# FOOD, DRUGS, AND AGING

**Ruth E. Dunkle, Ph.D.,** received her doctorate in the Social Sciences and her M.S.W. from Syracuse University. She taught at the School of Social Work at San Diego State University and the School of Applied Social Sciences at Case Western Reserve University before joining the faculty of the School of Social Work at the University of Michigan. Her research interests and publications have been in the areas of mental health, language impairment of the elderly, and service utilization for impaired elders. She is co-author of *The Older Aphasic Person: Strategies in Treatment and Diagnosis* and co-editor of *Communications Technology and the Elderly: Issues and Forecasts.*

**Grace J. Petot, M.S., R.D.,** is a registered dietitian and Assistant Professor of Nutrition and of Epidemiology and Biostatistics in the School of Medicine at Case Western Reserve University. Upon receiving her B.S. in Food Science at Michigan State University, she worked for the food industry in research and development of food products. She received her M.S. in Nutrition at Case Western Reserve University, where she presently teaches undergraduate courses in Food Science and Dietary Patterns and a graduate course in Nutrition for the Aging and Aged. Research interests include computerization of food composition tables, methods for determining food intake, and dietary patterns of the elderly.

**Amasa B. Ford, M.D.,** received his medical degree from Harvard Medical School and trained in internal medicine at Massachusetts General Hospital and University Hospitals of Cleveland. From 1954 to 1969 he was on the staff of Benjamin Rose Hospital in Cleveland, Ohio (geriatrics), where he served as Medical Director from 1960 to 1969. He is currently Professor of Epidemiology and Biostatistics, Family Medicine, and Medicine and Associate Dean for Geriatric Medicine, all at the Case Western Reserve University School of Medicine. Dr. Ford has done research in heart disease, geriatrics, work physiology, health services, and epidemiological aspects of community health. He is the author of *The Doctor's Perspective on Urban Health in America* and is co-editor of three recent books, *The Practice of Geriatric Medicine, Suicide in Children and Adolescents,* and *The Physical and Mental Health of Aged Women.*

# Food, Drugs, and Aging

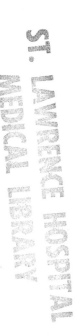

Ruth E. Dunkle, Ph.D.
Grace J. Petot, M.S., R.D.
Amasa B. Ford, M.D.
*Editors*

SPRINGER PUBLISHING COMPANY
New York

Springer Publishing Company, Inc.
536 Broadway
New York, NY 10012

86 87 88 89 90 / 5 4 3 2 1

---

Library of Congress Cataloging-in-Publication Data

Food, drugs, and aging.

    Edited versions of papers presented at a symposium
held in the fall of 1984 in Cleveland, Ohio and
sponsored by the Center on Aging and Health at
Case Western Reserve University.
    Bibliography: p.
    Includes index.
    1. Geriatric pharmacology—Congresses.  2. Aged—
Nutrition—Congresses.  I. Dunkle, Ruth E.  II. Petot,
Grace J.  III. Ford, Amasa B.
RC953.7.F64   1986      615'.1'0880565      86-22044
ISBN 0-8261-5050-0

---

Printed in the United States of America

# Contents

# Contributors

**Karl E. Anderson, M.D.,** Director, Clinical Research Center, and Professor of Medicine, New York Medical College, Valhalla, NY.

**Dorothy Booth, Ph.D., R.N.,** Assistant Professor, College of Nursing, Wayne State University, Detroit, MI.

**Ronni Chernoff, Ph.D., R.D.,** Associate Director, Geriatric Research Education and Clinical Center, John L. McClellan Memorial Veterans' Hospital, Little Rock, AR.

**Bess Dana, M.S.S.A.,** Professor of Community Medicine, Department of Community Medicine, The Mount Sinai School of Medicine, New York, NY.

**Jacqueline Dunbar, Ph.D., R.N.,** Assistant Professor in Psychiatry, Epidemiology and Nursing and Director of Nursing, Western Psychiatric Institute and Clinic, Pittsburgh, PA.

**Linda A. Hershey, M.D., Ph.D.,** Assistant Professor of Neurology and Medicine, Case Western Reserve University School of Medicine and University Hospitals of Cleveland, Cleveland, OH.

**Cary S. Kart, Ph.D.,** Professor of Sociology and Chair, Department of Sociology, Anthropology and Social Work, University of Toledo, Toledo, OH.

**Lois Kramer, B.A., R.D.,** Consulting Dietician, Metabolic Section, Veterans Administration Hospital, Hines, IL.

**Patricia McCormack, MRCPI, DCH,** Lecturer in Therapeutics, Department of Clinical Pharmacology, Royal College of Surgeons in Ireland, Dublin.

**Michael N. Mulvilhill, Dr.P.H.,** Associate Professor of Community Medicine, Department of Community Medicine, The Mount Sinai School of Medicine, New York, NY.

**Kevin O'Malley, M.D., Ph.D.,** Professor, Clinical Pharmacology, Royal College of Surgeons in Ireland, Dublin.

**Dace Osis,** Supervisor, Chemistry Laboratory, Metabolic Section, Veterans Administration Hospital, Hines, IL.

**Joseph G. Ouslander, M.D.,** Assistant Professor of Medicine, Division of Geriatric Medicine, UCLA School of Medicine; Medical Director, Nursing Home Care Unit, Veterans Administration Medical Center, Sepulveda, CA.

**Richard S. Rivlin, M.D.,** Chief, Nutrition Service, Memorial Sloan-Kettering Cancer Center and Professor of Medicine and Chief, Nutrition Division, New York Hospital-Cornell Medical Center, New York, NY.

**Nathan W. Shock, Ph.D.,** Scientist Emeritus, Gerontology Research Center, National Institute on Aging, Francis Scott Key Medical Center, Baltimore, MD.

**Herta Spencer, M.D.,** Chief, Metabolic Section, Veterans Administration Hospital, Hines, IL.

**Donald M. Watkin, M.D., M.P.H., F.A.C.P.,** Research Professor of Medicine, Department of Medicine, School of Medicine and Health Sciences, The George Washington University, Washington, DC.

**Ann L. Whall, Ph.D., R.N., F.A.A.N.,** Professor, School of Nursing, University of Michigan, Ann Arbor, MI.

# Preface

For older persons in America, food and drugs can be sources of comfort as well as pain. The nutritional needs of many adults change significantly after the age of 70, and their special dietary needs are little understood. Having the ability to purchase food and drugs to sustain life does not ensure their safe and effective use. Drugs can influence the dietary intake of nutrients and their utilization and elimination. On the other hand, the person's nutritional status can affect the efficacy and toxicity of drug treatment. This multifaceted issue of food and drugs is further complicated by the social, cultural, and economic condition of the older American. Knowledge in these areas has not kept pace with the increasing number and proportion of older persons in the United States, many of whom require therapeutic regimens.

There has been little emphasis on the biomedical relationship of drugs and food among older people, nor has the relationship been adequately explored from social, political, or psychological viewpoints. Age-related physiological changes in the gastrointestinal tract, in body composition, in metabolism, and in excretion all compound the problem of drug effectiveness in the elderly. Pharmacokinetics can be altered further by such factors as the older person's reduced activity, confinement to bed, dehydration, congestive heart failure, and thyroid disease. Similarly, age factors affect the dietary intake of nutrients and their absorption and metabolism. Malnutrition can result from disease states or decreased dietary intake. Certain physical disabilities, restricted income, health and dental problems, and social isolation can contribute to a poor state of nutrition. Drug–diet interrelationships, though subtle, can have significant effects on the older person's well-being. More important, few studies have considered how elderly patients can help themselves and what their physicians can do to gain awareness of these potential problems and effect practical solutions.

A major purpose of this book is to present the interrelationship of food and drugs for the elderly within a biomedical and social perspective. The older person is viewed as an active participant in the successful development of a drug–nutrient regime. This volume consists of edited versions of papers presented at a symposium, "Food, Drugs, and Aging," held in the Fall of 1984 in Cleveland, Ohio, and sponsored by the University Center on Aging and Health at Case Western Reserve University. The introductory chapter, *Issues in Nutrition, Pharmacology, and Aging,* brings together information on physiological changes associated with aging; the role of nutrition in deterring or abating health hazards associated with aging such as coronary artery disease, hypertension, osteoporosis, and cancer; and the effect of nutrition for prevention of side effects caused by drugs. Richard S. Rivlin, Chief of Nutrition Services at Memorial Sloan-Kettering Cancer Center, explores the metabolism of hormones, drugs, and nutritional agents. While emphasizing the role of nutrition as a therapeutic agent, he cautions that it may not be the sole treatment measure.

In Part I, *Issues in Pharmacology,* McCormack and O'Malley cover biological and medical aspects of drug treatment in the elderly. These physicians also take into account the socioeconomic, physiological, and pathological context of effective drug utilization in the body as they examine pharmacodynamic responses and pharmacokinetic properties of drugs. Ouslander warns against the hazards of polypharmacy in the elderly: Adverse drug reactions, drug–drug interactions, drug–patient interactions, poor compliance, and increased costs coalesce in the older population to make drug usage problematic. Dana and Mulvilhill enlarge on the social perspective of drug therapy as they examine social and environmental characteristics affecting the older population and point out the virtual nonexistence of a health care model capable of integrating the social prescription and the drug regimen.

Part II, *Issues in Nutrition,* focuses on the relationship of diseases and nutrition as affected by social, cultural, and economic concerns of older people. Watkin, unlike Rivlin, describes nutrition as the primary therapeutic agent in the prevention and treatment of most major causes of disability and reviews food components such as fat, carbohydrates, and protein for their therapeutic benefit. Spencer, Kramer, and Osis narrow their comments to one specific nutritionally related health concern for older persons: bone loss. After identifying osteoporosis in elderly women as a major public health problem, they explore the associated diagnostic and treatment concerns. Kart's paper shifts the focus from the biomedical aspects of nutrition to the social and cultural aspects that produce nutritional vulnerability among the aged. The last paper of this section, written by Hershey, deals with the nonscientific dimensions of food and drug use fads. Her historical perspective provides a glimpse into the emotional and social components of food and drugs.

The concluding segment of this text, Part III, *Introduction to Drug–Nutrient Interaction,* highlights the therapeutic issues related to drugs and nutrition. The stage is set by Shock, who describes age decrements in performance, noting the variability in different organ systems within the same individual. Anderson's review of changes in the enzyme systems that metabolize drugs, hormones, and other chemicals that can alter the response of the older person is complemented by Chernoff's chapter on nutrition and chemotherapy in the elderly. Chernoff examines the effects of cancer and then chemotherapy on the nutritional status of the older cancer victim. Whall and Booth view nutrition and polypharmacy in a specific environmental context, the institution. Their practical approach underscores the significant impact drugs and food have on the quality of life for many older people. The book concludes with Dunbar's examination of compliance of older persons with diet and drug prescriptions. Strategies to aid the professional and elder in dealing with problems of compliance are suggested.

With the increasing population and number of elderly people in the United States, knowledge of nutrition and drug use needs to expand. While substantial data have been generated in animals, only limited information exists as to the significance and frequency of drug–diet–nutrient interactions among the elderly. This book offers health care professionals and other service providers, as well as the elderly and their families, a synopsis of our progress toward acquiring the information necessary to sustain life through the use of drugs and food in a more successful and satisfying fashion.

**RED**

**GJP**

**ABF**

# Introduction

# Issues in Nutrition, Pharmacology, and Aging

*Richard S. Rivlin*

Food, drugs, and aging are universal concerns because we all eat, we all grow older, and as we grow older we use increasing numbers of drugs. In fact, it is the aging population—which uses the largest number of drugs, uses them for the most prolonged period of time and for a variety of reasons—that is most likely to suffer from the ill effects of drug therapy. Our challenge as physicians and scientists is to learn how to use nutrition to prevent disease, how to slow the process of aging, and how to make drug use more effective and less harmful, particularly in the elderly population.

The first goal of food and nutrition should be to prevent disease so that drugs will not be needed at all. Food is actually a medicine and it is also a drug, because individual nutrients in food have specific actions. Our next goal should be to use nutrition wisely, once disease has developed and drugs are needed for treatment. We must learn how to use nutrition to improve the therapeutic efficacy of drugs, to enable them to be

This research was supported by grants 5PO1 CA 29502, 5T32 CA 09427, and CA 08748 from the National Institutes of Health and by grants from the Stella and Charles Guttman Foundation, the William H. Donner Foundation, Inc., the Alcoholic Beverage Medical Research Foundation, the Richard Molin Memorial Foundation, the Loet A. Velmans Fund, and the General Foods Fund. This research was performed in the Sperry Corporation Nutrition Research Laboratory.

3

prescribed for shorter periods of time, and to minimize their side effects.

It is of interest that the elderly are predisposed to three times the incidence of adverse drug effects than are persons below 50 years of age (Judge & Caird, 1978). To some extent this finding reflects greater usage of drugs, but it also indicates increased vulnerability. Nutritional depletion due to drugs usually develops gradually and results from the cumulative effects of prolonged therapy, frequently escaping the physician's attention.

Much of the need for drugs and the problems associated with their usage would be minimized if enough effort were given to the proper use of nutrition in the prevention of disease, particularly heart disease, cancer, renal disease, diabetes, and osteoporosis.

## THE POTENTIAL OF NUTRITION FOR THE PREVENTION OF DISEASE

At the present time many of the most important diseases in the United States appear to have a nutritional component to their pathogenesis, knowledge of which may be helpful in their prevention. It may be useful to review some of the recent highlights in this field.

### Heart Disease

Much evidence now indicates that nutrition may play an important role in the development of several different kinds of heart disease. With respect to atherosclerosis, there are now findings that the prevalence of heart disease is directly correlated with the serum cholesterol level and that a lowering of the serum cholesterol is associated with a decrease in the prevalence of heart attacks. There also appears to be an association between the prevalence of heart disease and the serum triglyceride level, which also has a major dietary component.

Salt intake has also been recognized as a correlate of hypertension, both from country to country and within certain populations in a single country. Particular individuals, nevertheless, are much more susceptible to the hypertension-causing effects of salt than are others.

Another dietary nutrient importantly related to heart disease is alcohol. There is now evidence that hypertension is significantly increased in prevalence in individuals who consume large amounts of alcohol. It had been believed that having one to two drinks daily would raise the HDL component of serum cholesterol and thereby might actually be beneficial for heart disease. Later studies, however, have generally been less enthusiastic about the efficacy of this practice. Furthermore, alcohol in large doses is a cause of cardiomyopathy, an infiltrative form of heart disease.

Another nutrient that has recently received attention in relation to hypertension is calcium. There are now suggestive observations that in some persons a high-calcium diet, or supplementation with calcium, may result in lowering of high blood pressure (McCarron, Morris, & Cole, 1982). It is important to realize that a diet high in salt tends to result in greater loss of calcium in the urine and that, conversely, a diet low in salt results in calcium retention. Thus, the efficacy of calcium upon reducing blood pressure may possibly be related to the concomitant dietary intake of salt. Serum magnesium has also been related to the renin-angiotensin, aldosterone system and to the regulation of hypertension (Resnick, Laragh, Sealey, & Alderman, 1983).

Investigations in China indicate that deficiency of selenium may be a very significant factor in the etiology of Keshan Disease, a rare form of heart disease. Other examples show that there is a relationship between specific nutrients and heart disease and hypertension.

## Cancer

There is now increasing evidence that the prevalence of various cancers among nations around the world is importantly related to certain components of the diet. A diet high in fat has been associated with an increase in cancer of the breast, prostate and colon and other malignancies. In those countries of the world that have little dietary fat, such as Thailand, breast cancer, prostate cancer, and colon cancer are very rare. By contrast, in the Netherlands and Denmark, which have among the highest intakes of dietary fat, the prevalence of these cancers is very great (Graham & Mettlin, 1979; Reddy et al., 1980). The relation of fat to cancer is obviously a complex subject, but on balance, the predominance of evidence would suggest that it is reasonable to consider reducing our dietary intake of fat as a possible means of prevention of these cancers. This measure would be most appropriate for those individuals who are at highest risk for breast cancer, such as women who have had a previous breast malignancy or those who have a very high family history of breast cancer.

Another nutrient that appears to be importantly related to the development of cancer is vitamin A and its retinoid derivatives, including beta carotene. It appears now that a decrease in the dietary intake of vitamin A and/or beta carotene may result in an increased prevalence of certain epithelial cancers, particularly cancer of the lung (Mettlin, Graham, & Swanson, 1979). The protective effect of previous dietary intake of beta carotene and/or vitamin A upon the prevalence of lung cancer seems to be most apparent in those persons who are heavy smokers (Mettlin, Graham, & Swanson, 1979). Unfortunately, measurements of the serum levels of vitamin A have not proven to be effective as a means of prediction of cancer risk. This observation may be a reflection of the fact that the serum levels of vitamin A tend in general to be in a relatively narrow range and to be a poor reflection of long-term dietary intake.

The subject of diet and cancer is, of course, very involved, and one should at least mention that there may be possible effects of selenium, magnesium, nitrites, fiber, vitamin C, zinc, and other nutrients. This discussion only serves to point out that certain common nutrients may influence the development of specific cancers (Rivlin, 1982). Obviously this is an area of great scientific interest, and more research is vitally needed.

## Diabetes

It is widely recognized that the best oral agent for both the prevention and treatment of diabetes is a good diet. Diet is important in maintaining body weight, in delaying the onset of atherosclerosis, and in maintaining electrolyte balance, in addition to keeping the blood sugar levels within the normal range. Indeed, no discussion of diabetes would be complete without mentioning that the diet is the most important method of approaching diabetes in general.

Within the past few years there is increasing enthusiasm for a diet high in fiber and complex carbohydrates, which, if properly chosen, may help to keep the blood sugar in a more even range throughout the day, delay and spread out the rise in insulin levels in response to food, and altogether make diabetic management easier to achieve under ordinary circumstances (Jovanovic & Peterson, 1985).

## Renal Diseases

The loss of kidney function with age is a well-recognized phenomenon. The glomerular filtration rate decreases at approximately .5 to 1 percent per year, starting from early adult life. As a result of the loss of renal function, elderly subjects are more susceptible to the side effects of drugs, since they have a delay in drug excretion and a diminished ability to respond to changes in acid/base balance (Masoro, 1976). There is now evidence from animal model systems and to a lesser extent from human studies that a diet low in protein may delay the onset of renal disease due to aging and that, in patients with chronic renal disease, may delay its progression. Other components of one's diet, such as phosphate, calcium, sodium, and zinc may also be expected to influence certain features of renal disease.

## Osteoporosis

Efforts to prevent the bone loss associated with aging are now focused on diet, together with exercise and female hormones. Now there is widespread agreement that the single most important dietary factor is calcium, an element that is consumed in inadequate amounts by a distressingly large proportion of American women (Heaney et al., 1982). Contemporary strategies are now aimed at increasing calcium intake early in life, in order to make peak bone mass as high as possible, and then maintaining calcium intake throughout adult life in order to delay the onset of bone loss that occurs after the age of 25 to 35, and particularly following menopause, when the rate of bone loss is greatest.

Calcium is not, however, the only dietary nutrient involved in osteoporosis, as vitamin D facilitates the intestinal absorption of calcium and its mobilization from bone. Phosphate is an important component of bone matrix. Dietary salt may be relevant in that it regulates urinary calcium excretion, as noted already. There are reports that vitamin A may accelerate bone loss of aging (Navia & Harris, 1980). The possible effects of vitamin C require clarification. Since chronic acidosis of any etiology tends to mobilize calcium from bone, there may be possible complications from long-term use of megadoses of vitamin C. Dietary fiber makes calcium less bioavailable, and dietary zinc in large amounts decreases calcium absorption. Other nutrient-nutrient interactions have potential implications for osteoporosis.

In summary, it is increasingly apparent that, with respect to some major causes of mortality and morbidity in the United States, namely, cancer, heart disease, diabetes, renal disease, and osteoporosis, nutritional measures should be strongly considered as a possible means of prevention. These issues are highly complex but hold great promise for the future and urgently require further research.

## THE POTENTIAL OF NUTRITION FOR PREVENTION OF SIDE EFFECTS CAUSED BY DRUGS

### General Considerations

Just as the concept of risk factors has been useful in understanding the development of heart disease, similar attention should be directed toward elucidating possible risk factors for the development of malnutrition. These factors would include use of multiple drugs, alcoholism, malabsorption, and other items. It is essential to realize that elderly people may be vulnerable to the nutritional side effects of drugs if they are already in a marginal nutritional status. There is certainly abundant evidence that many elderly individuals are in a marginal nutritional status as a result of poverty, physical isolation, reduced mobility, depression, and illness, as well as a number of other reasons (Rivlin, 1981). We now recognize that drug-induced nutritional deficiencies that commonly occur in older individuals are seldom recognized and are often preventable.

Probably the categories of drugs that most frequently cause clinically significant malnutrition in older subjects are diuretics and laxatives. These agents are often taken for prolonged periods of time by vulnerable individuals. Laxatives tend to accelerate gastrointestinal transit time and to result in excessive loss of nutrients due to diminished intestinal absorption. When mineral oil and other fat-soluble agents are taken as laxatives, they may dissolve the fat-soluble vitamins—namely, A, D, E, and K—and result in their increased loss through the stool. Diuretics will cause urinary potassium loss, as is well known, but also that of zinc, copper, magnesium, and other elements (Hathcock & Coon, 1978; Roe, 1975).

## Effects of Drugs on Vitamin $B_2$ Metabolism

In an effort to elucidate some of the factors that regulate vitamin metabolism, our laboratory has been exploring those hormones, nutrients, and drugs that regulate the metabolism of vitamin $B_2$. It is not widely appreciated that vitamin $B_2$, or riboflavin, shares certain structural features with a number of clinically used psychotropic agents, including chlorpromazine, a phenothiazine derivative, and the tricyclic antidepressants, imipramine and amitriptyline. These considerations prompted us to determine whether drugs of these two categories act as riboflavin antagonists, inhibiting the formation of flavin adenine dinucleotide (FAD) from riboflavin. Our studies over a period of years have shown that phenothiazine derivatives and tricyclic antidepressants do inhibit riboflavin metabolism markedly, both *in vitro* and *in vivo* (Pinto, Huang, & Rivlin, 1981). Furthermore, chlorpromazine impairs thyroxine stimulation of FAD formation (Pinto, Huang, & Rivlin, 1985). Recent observations indicate that riboflavin metabolism in cardiac tissue is particularly sensitive to tricyclic antidepressants (Pinto,

Huang, Pelliccione, & Rivlin, 1982). Psychotropic drugs that are structurally unrelated to riboflavin do not inhibit flavin formation in heart, liver, cerebrum, or cerebellum.

Inasmuch as these psychotropic drugs are widely used clinically and furthermore because many patients have only marginally adequate nutritional status, we have been concerned that serious drug-induced riboflavin deficiency may occur in this setting. In an animal model, significant depletion of tissue FAD tends to occur following treatment with low doses of chlorpromazine, and the rate of development of riboflavin deficiency can be accelerated by treatment with this drug. These findings in their entirety underscore the need to direct attention toward the nutritional side effects of drugs, particularly when therapy is prolonged and nutritional status precarious.

Other studies now in progress explore the effect of adriamycin, a widely used anticancer drug, on inhibiting vitamin $B_2$ metabolism. This drug also has a number of structural similarities to vitamin $B_2$.

Alcohol causes riboflavin deficiency, which may develop as a result of a poor diet or possibly because of specific effects of ethanol upon $B_2$ metabolism. Preliminary indications are that alcohol inhibits both riboflavin absorption from the intestinal tract and the degradation of food FAD to riboflavin, which is necessary prior to absorption. If this finding is confirmed and extended, it would suggest that food sources of riboflavin may be particularly vulnerable to alcohol ingestion and that therapy of alcoholic patients may perhaps be more effective initially with pure vitamins rather than with food sources of vitamin $B_2$.

## SUMMARY AND CONCLUSION

It is apparent from this brief review that much has been learned about food, drugs, and aging but much more remains to be uncovered. The conversion of dietary vitamins to active coenzyme derivatives represents an important control point in intermediary metabolism for hormones, drugs, and nutritional factors. We must continue our efforts to elucidate how drugs interfere with nutritional status and be aware of those nutritional practices that may make patients vulnerable to the side effects of drugs.

We also must have realistic expectations as to what nutrition can do. Nutrition cannot reverse the aging process, nor can it give super energy. Nutrition should be viewed as an adjunct to any treatment plan and not as its replacement. It is a tragedy when appropriate pharmacologic agents are discarded for the illusory benefits of megadoses of vitamins and minerals. Thus, important as nutrition is, it must not be regarded as the sole means of therapy or prevention of disease when other measures are more effective.

# Part I
# Issues in
# Pharmacology

# Introduction

Pharmacology reaches beyond the knowledge of the physiological effects of drugs to include a complete view of treatment: medical, social, and psychological. These perspectives, as related to the elderly, are reviewed in the following three chapters. Although utilizing widely different views, these authors acknowledge the complex nature of drug treatment of the old.

In Chapter 1, McCormack and O'Malley, of the Department of Clinical Pharmacology, Royal College of Surgeons in Ireland, focus on the socioeconomic, physiological, and pathological changes that accompany aging and that affect the body's use of drugs. Raising the issue of multiple pathology with increasing age, they set the stage for a discussion of the effect of disease on the pharmacokinetic behavior and pharmacodynamic responses of the older person to therapeutic agents.

Pharmacokinetics refers to processes such as absorption, distribution, metabolism, and excretion, which affect the impact that drugs have on the human body. While there is little change in the absorption and metabolism of drugs in older persons, distribution, especially of single doses of drugs, is likely to be altered, as is the excretion of the drug due to declining renal function. Pharmacodynamics of drug therapies, although related to pharmacokinetic factors, are independent and typically receptor mediated. A discussion ensues of the responsiveness and affinity in the elderly of receptors for various types of drugs. A general approach to prescribing drugs for this age group concludes this chapter, thus leaving the reader with a well-grounded understanding of the biological and medical aspects of successful drug treatment in the elderly.

Ouslander's discussion of polypharmacy and the elderly in Chapter 2 adds another dimension to the reader's understanding of pharmacology. With 12% of the population over 65 years of age availing themselves of more than one quarter of the prescribed drugs, the elderly are likely candidates for adverse drug responses due to drug-drug interactions or drug-patient interactions. The physician's attitude and behavior, as well as the older patient's expectations of drug use, further complicate the nature of response. Certainly poor compliance cannot be overlooked as a potential result of polypharmacy. The prescription of multiple drugs in complicated dosing regimens and increasing drug costs exacerbate the problem of noncompliance. Ouslander concludes his chapter on a practical note by specifying the necessary procedures to ensure avoidance of the hazards of polypharmacy: educating health professionals, especially physicians, about altering their prescribing habits, and informing the public.

In the final chapter of this section, Dana and Mulvilhill explore the social perspective of pharmacology of older people by identifying social and psychological factors that are implicated in drug problems and recommending solutions in the educational and delivery system of social health services. Demonstrating that both the elderly patient and the physician contribute to the drug-taking behavior of the patient, the authors help the reader appreciate the complex nature of adverse drug reactions among the elderly. Multiple issues—such as the prescribing behavior of the physician, unclear rules for drug usage, noncompliance, and multiple drug use, as well as social factors of social isolation, low self-esteem, and apathy—emerge as risk factors for the negative therapeutic outcome of drug treatment.

Few social health models exist as guides to the solution of health problems. Dana and Mulvilhill note only one, the health decision model, which reflects patient preferences, needed knowledge, and social interaction factors. Still missing in this model is consideration of organizational characteristics, payment mechanisms, eligibility requirements, and social provisions of the provider and consumer. This chapter ends with a clear warning that professional self-interests are a major obstacle to implementing a social health model. Values and knowledge of the social needs and rights of the older patient are necessary if the model is to be useful.

**R.E.D.**

# 1

# Biological and Medical Aspects of Drug Treatment in the Elderly

*Patricia McCormack*
*Kevin O'Malley*

Elderly patients comprise 12 percent of the population in Western countries (Giannetti, 1983) and use more than one quarter of all prescriptions dispensed. Furthermore, the elderly appear to be more susceptible to adverse drug reactions than younger patients and differ in drug handling and responsiveness as well (Bender, 1974; Lasagna, 1956; Schmucker, 1984; Siegel, 1982). This is due in part to the fact that the number of therapeutic agents utilized increases with age. Accordingly, it behooves the practitioner to identify the elderly as a special group of patients and individualize therapeutic regimens with these issues in mind.

In this chapter we will consider (1) variables that may be responsible for altering responsiveness to drugs, (2) adverse drug reactions that seem to be age dependent, and (3) compliance with drug therapy. Specifically, we will consider pharmacokinetic properties and pharmacodynamic responses in relation to aging and we will suggest a general approach to prescribing drugs for older persons.

# GENERAL CONSIDERATIONS

The elderly form a highly heterogenous group of patients ranging from completely independent, mobile, physically active
persons to those with serious debilitating disease. Bearing this
variability in mind, let us consider some of the differences
between older persons and their younger counterparts that influence drug use.

## *Differential Responsiveness*

Variables altering responsiveness may be of a social or physical
nature. Multiple pathology in older persons predicts an increase
in the number of drugs that a patient is likely to be given and
increases the likelihood of adverse drug reactions and of unwanted drug interactions. Diseases may alter the pharmacokinetic behavior and pharmacodynamic responses of the patient
to these therapeutic agents. Certain physical ailments may predict certain types of treatment as well. For instance, arthritis
may make it more difficult for older persons to manipulate an
inhaler, small tablets, or "childproof" containers. Old people
with poor eyesight may not be able to administer precise doses
of insulin or correctly identify medication.

## *Environments*

Environments such as institutions may have an important influence on drug consumption. Prescribing is often done by nonspe-
cialists, and "as required" orders are frequent. Where there is
understaffing and inadequate supervision, errors in prescribing
can readily occur. Furthermore, the unwanted effects of drugs
may go unnoticed until they present as a major health problem.

## *Patterns of Drug Prescribing*

There is a higher rate of prescribing of hypnotics and laxatives
in the elderly. As the elderly have an increased susceptibility
to infection (Makinodan, James, Inamizu, & Chang, 1984;

Oyeyinka, 1984), the increased level of antibiotic prescriptions may be justified. Great care is required when prescribing particular groups of antimicrobials (i.e., aminoglycosides), due to their higher incidence of toxicity in elderly patients (Yoshikawa, 1984).

## PHARMACOKINETICS

The term *pharmacokinetics* refers to the various processes whereby drugs are handled in the body: absorption, distribution, metabolism, and excretion. There are a number of well-described changes in pharmacokinetics in the elderly (Balant, 1984; Crooks & Stevenson, 1981). We will consider the four pharmacokinetic processes individually.

### Absorption

There is a decrease in many aspects of gastrointestinal functioning in the elderly; however, this does not appear to be reflected in clinically significant changes in the rate or extent of drug absorption in this age group.

### Distribution

With advancing age there are changes in body composition. For example, body fat increases as a proportion of body weight, and total body water decreases. In broad terms this means that those drugs distributed into body fat tend to have an increased volume of distribution, whereas those that tend to be confined to body water have a decreased volume of distribution. For example, diazepam is relatively fat soluble and is distributed in fat to a large extent. As age increases, the half-life of the drug (the amount of time it takes the body's mechanisms for biotransformation and excretion to decrease the plasma concentration of a drug by 50%) increases; this results in an extremely long duration of chemical action in old people. In general, the decrease in lean body mass and total body water result in an increase in plasma levels of water-soluble drugs such as ethanol, and a decrease in lipid-soluble drugs (Williams, 1984). In the very old the levels of all drugs would tend to be higher for a given dose. Serum albumen diminishes with age and as a consequence so do the number of binding sites for albumen-bound drugs (Upton, Williams, Kelly, & Jones, 1984). With single doses of drugs there will be an increase in free fraction, and this may result in greater effect. However, with chronic drug use, the amount of free drug in the plasma tends to remain unchanged. Total drug levels are slightly diminished, and one would predict that the intensity and duration of pharmacological effect would be unaltered.

*Metabolism*

The rate of drug metabolism varies enormously from person to person. Determinants of metabolic rate include genetic and environmental factors, concurrent drug therapy, physical status as well as age. In general, enzyme systems such as metabolic pathways in the liver seem to be less efficient with increasing age (Gershon, 1979; Okada & Dice, 1984). Factors other than age, however, seem to be more important determinants of drug metabolism in the elderly (Feely, Pereira, Guy, & Hockings, 1984; Sambuy & Bittles, 1984; Vestal, 1978). There is no age-related change in acetylation (hydralazine and isoniazid). Enzyme induction can occur but perhaps not to the same extent as in younger patients (Cusack, Kelly, Lavan, Noel, & O'Malley, 1980; Twum-Barima, Finnigan, Habash, Cape, & Carruthers, 1984).

After absorption, drugs go to the liver, and many are extracted from the blood before actually getting to the systemic circulation. This is variously referred to as the first-pass effect, first-pass metabolism, or presystemic elimination of drugs. The first-pass effect is more efficient in the young than in the old. In other words, there is a diminution in the ability of the older liver to extract drugs on the first pass through the liver; therefore, more of the drug gets to the systemic circulation, with enhanced drug effect usually the result.

*Excretion*

Renal function declines with age (Hollenberg et al., 1974; Shock, 1952). The glomerular filtration rate is reduced by 35% from the ages 20 to 90 years. Reduction also occurs in renal plasma flow, urine concentration ability, and sodium conservation. The circadian diurnal rhythm of ADH secretion also appears to be reversed, resulting in increasing nocturia, which may be worsened or provoked by diuretic drugs. The overall result of declining renal function is a decrease in the rate of elimination of renally excreted drugs and thus a prolongation of half life. Important drugs in this regard include digoxin and the aminoglycoside antibiotics. In clinical practice the dose of these drugs must be decreased to take into account the reduced rate of elimination.

This is also particularly important with drugs having a narrow therapeutic ratio. Digoxin is an extremely toxic drug. If one inadvertently gives the standard dose (based on appraisals for a young person) to an elderly person, toxicity might well ensue. This applies as well to the aminoglycocides and probably to cimetidine. It does not apply to penicillin because the serious adverse effects of penicillin are not related to dose. It really makes very little difference if one uses a million units of penicillin or 10 million; it has a very wide therapeutic rate.

## PHARMACODYNAMICS

Certain drugs have been shown to produce either a greater or lesser response in elderly patients, independent of pharmacokinetic factors (Crooks, 1983b). Most responses are receptor mediated; hence, interest has been focused on receptor function in humans, animals, and cell lines (Hayflick, 1980, 1984; Holliday, Huschtscha, Tarrant, & Kirkwood, 1977; Ito, 1979; Roth & Hess, 1982). Particular interest has been directed toward responsiveness, numbers, and affinity of receptors.

Beta-adrenoceptor-mediated responses provide an interesting example of receptor function (Fitzgerald, Doyle, Kelly, & O'Malley, 1984; Kelly & O'Malley, 1984). The heart rate response to isoprenaline is reduced in the elderly (Vestal, Wood, & Shand,

1979). Initially, it was thought that beta-receptor numbers were diminished with age (Schocken & Roth, 1977), but it is now generally accepted that total receptor numbers are not significantly altered (Kelly & O'Malley, 1984). However, high-affinity receptors are reduced in the elderly (Feldman, Limbird, Nadeau, Robertson, & Wood, 1984). These findings appear to have clinical relevance in that responses to beta blockers are reduced with age. Furthermore, the beta-2 agonist effects of bronchodilators are reduced in the elderly (Ullah, Newman, & Saunders, 1981).

Explanations that have been offered for the reduced response in the elderly include higher circulating levels of noradrenaline, causing down-regulation of high-affinity receptors. On the other hand, there is evidence that there may be changes downstream from the beta adrenoceptor, and Kelly and O'Malley (1984) have hypothesized that, with aging, all membrane components have restrictive effects on adenylate cyclase activity. Thus, more than one mechanism may be operating. Much of the beta-receptor research has been done using white blood cells, both polymorphonuclear cells and lymphocytes. The *in vitro* findings remain to be confirmed in other cells.

Reduced responses to steroid hormones with age also have been shown in various tissues (Kalimi & Seifler, 1979; Rosner & Cristofalo, 1981; Sapolsky, Krey, & McEwen, 1983). This relates to reduction in the number of specific glucocorticoid receptor binding sites, with no change in their affinity, and may have clinical relevance with regard to glucocorticoid-influenced functions in the limbus, which (in rats) demonstrate deficits with age.

In contrast to this, elderly patients often have increased responses to various psychotropic drugs. Benzodiazepines produce varying responses, in that some have an increased effect in the elderly whereas in others there is no change in response. There is a pharmacokinetic basis for some (Klotz, Avant, Hoyumpa, Schenker, & Wilkinson, 1975) but not all (Reidenberg et al., 1978) of these changes. There is no pharmacokinetic explanation for the increased effects of nitrazepam in elderly patients (Castleden, George, Marcer, & Hallett, 1977; Swift, Swift, Hamley, Stevenson, & Crooks, 1983), and altered pharmacodynamic responses are a more likely explanation. No differences were observed in the response to lorezepam or oxazepam in the elderly.

Animal experiments indicate increased responses to haloperidol (Campbell & Baldessarini, 1981). Ethanol produces increased drowsiness in elderly persons, independently of pharmacokinetic variables (Poikolainen, 1984; Vestal, 1978). Several authors agree that the elderly are more susceptible to the anticholinergic side effects of a variety of drugs, such as tricyclic antidepressants and phenothiazines (Jarvik & Kakkar, 1981; Veith, 1984). Studies in animals (mice and rats) suggest that there are reduced numbers of muscarinic receptors (Avissar, Egozi, & Sokolovsky, 1981; Burchinsky, 1984; Lippa et al., 1981) and GABA receptors (Calderini et al., 1981) with age.

From a clinical point of view there is a high incidence of tardive dyskinesia in elderly patients on chronic neuroleptic therapy (Smith & Baldessarini, 1980). This is also more frequently seen in elderly patients taking metaclopramide (Orme & Tallis, 1984). While the cause of this is complex, it is reasonable to suggest an interplay of the four postulated receptor subtypes (Burchinsky, 1984).

Other drugs also have been shown to have increased responses. These include lignocaine, which has twice the incidence of toxicity in elderly patients; warfarin (Kelley & O'Malley, 1979; O'Malley, Stevenson, Ward, Wood, & Crooks, 1977); halothane (Gregory, Eger, & Munson, 1969); and analgesics such as morphine sulphate (Bellville, Forrest, Miller, & Brown, 1971; Kaiko, 1980). In animals, the minimal effective plasma concentration of phenytoin is lower in old mice (Kitani et al., 1984).

Many drugs are more likely to produce confusion in the elderly, including nonsteroidal anti-inflammatory drugs, psychotropic agents, and tricyclic antidepressants. This could be related to increasing neuronal loss with age.

## HOMEOSTASIS

Loss of homeostatic responses is a hallmark of aging. Postural hypotension may be a special problem in elderly patients and is related to their reduced baroreceptor response to changes in blood pressure (McGarry et al., 1983). Similarly, altered thermal homeostasis puts the elderly at risk from certain drugs that interfere with temperature regulation, such as chlorpromazine (Collins & Exton-Smith 1983). The older person is less able to buffer perturbations in the physiological system, and, of course, physiological systems probably are perturbed more by drugs themselves than any other factor.

## ADVERSE DRUG REACTIONS

The elderly are three to seven times more susceptible than younger people to adverse drug reactions (Goldberg & Roberts, 1983). It seems likely that the principal contribution is from altered pharmacokinetics and polypharmacy. The number of adverse reactions doubles in 80-year-olds, compared with those in their fifth decade. Hurwitz (1969) found a similar but not as marked increase in adverse effects when comparing those over 60 to those less than 60 years of age.

## COMPLIANCE

Poor compliance is a practical problem with all prescriptions, in both young and old patients. Certain elderly patients are particularly at risk in this regard. Clearly those patients with poor eyesight, neurological deficit such as dementia or stroke, or arthritis may not comprehend instructions on the one hand or may be unable to comply for very good physical reasons on the other hand. It also may be true that the independent elderly are noncompliant as a result of adverse drug reactions. There is very good evidence that if you ask a person to take a drug more than twice a day, and if you ask a patient to take more than three different preparations, the level of compliance drops dramatically. While there may be theoretical reasons for giving all these drugs, in the majority of cases the drugs simply will not be taken. It is very chastening to realize that in some cases only about 50% of prescriptions are even filled, never mind taken.

## CONCLUSION

The elderly respond differently to certain types of drug therapy. These differences are quantitative rather than qualitative. The principles of prescribing remain essentially the same in young and old alike (Vestal, 1978). Individualization of drug therapy in this group requires an appreciation of the various changes they are experiencing and the ability to see each patient as being unique. Before prescribing, one should have a clear indication for a drug. Perhaps nondrug modalities may suffice. One must evaluate the patient, physically, psychologically, and socially; choose the minimum number of therapeutic agents; stop any drugs if possible; be aware of the pharmacological, pharmacokinetic, and pharmaceutical properties of each agent used; be aware of clinically significant interactions; and consider the cost and the likely benefit. Finally, it is important to review drug prescriptions frequently and to modify the regimen as required.

# 2
# Polypharmacy and the Elderly

*Joseph G. Ouslander*

To health professionals primarily involved in the care of the elderly, the problem of polypharmacy is no secret. An all too common scenario is played out in geriatric consultation clinics and specialized geriatric units every day: An elderly patient complains of any number of symptoms, many of which are severe and potentially disabling. Inspection of the bag full of drugs the patient has been taking reveals several prescribed by different physicians the patient has seen over recent months, each doctor often unaware of what the other physicians have prescribed. Also to be found are other over-the-counter nonprescription preparations and sometimes drugs the patient has borrowed from a relative or friend. It usually does not take long to determine the cause of the patients' symptoms.

Several surveys have documented that elderly persons in ambulatory-care settings, acute-care hospitals and long-term-care institutions are prescribed numerous drugs and drug doses (Kalchthaler, Coccaro, & Lichtiger, 1977; Lamy, 1980; May, Stewart, Hale, & Marks, 1982; Ray, Federspiel, & Schaffner, 1980; Reynolds, 1984; U.S. Senate, 1976). This polypharmacy in elderly persons has a number of implications, including a number of attendant hazards. These are:

Adverse drug reactions;
Drug–drug interactions;
Drug–patient interactions;
Poor compliance;
Increased costs to patients, institutions, and to the public.

The purpose of this chapter is to discuss these implications and hazards of polypharmacy in the elderly and to suggest strategies that will help minimize the problem.

## WHY IS THERE POLYPHARMACY?

Despite the hazards of polypharmacy, which are well known to most health professionals, the prescribing of multiple drugs for elderly persons is a persistent phenomenon. What underlies this practice, and can it be justified, given the problems it generates? While it is true that four out of five elderly persons have at least one chronic medical condition, many of these conditions can be managed without drug therapy. Elderly persons often present with numerous symptoms, and there is a tendency for physicians to prescribe a drug rather than attempt to determine the underlying cause of the symptom. This not only leads to inappropriate drug treatment and polypharmacy but can leave a potentially treatable problem undiagnosed (Kane, Ouslander, & Abrass, 1984; Ouslander, 1981). Occasionally drugs are prescribed to treat what are in fact symptoms caused by other drugs.

Physicians may prescribe drugs in this manner for several reasons. Most physicians have had no training in the care of elderly persons and find this patient population time consuming, frustrating, and difficult to care for. Fear of growing old, attribution of symptoms simply to old age, and other ageist attitudes add to this perspective. These attitudes are reinforced by caring for elderly persons in nursing homes, where patients are generally very disabled, physically unattractive, and have multiple incurable medical problems. Prescribing drugs can help physicians to feel they are at least doing something for their elderly patients.

Physician attitudes and behavior are not the only factors underlying polypharmacy. Ubiquitous and aggressive advertising and marketing of drugs certainly contributes to physician prescribing behavior (Avorn & Soumerai, 1983). Health professionals cannot read a journal, newsletter, or conference brochure without seeing a drug advertisement. Physicians are constantly bombarded by mail-order catalogs and drug salespeople pushing new or well-established products. Many patients add to this pressure by expecting and often demanding some type of drug therapy. Every physician has prescribed drugs against their better judgment, knowing that, if they did not, the patient would shop around until they found a doctor who would prescribe a drug. Rather than abandon the patient, increase the costs of care, and subject the patient to uncontrolled risks, many physicians succumb to this patient-generated pressure.

Thus, the roots of polypharmacy are multifactorial and not simply the result of ignorance on the part of prescribing health professionals. In order to minimize polypharmacy, each of the reasons we have discussed here must be confronted.

## THE HAZARDS OF POLYPHARMACY

### Adverse Drug Reactions

The most common and important consequence of polypharmacy is an increased risk of adverse drug reactions. The incidence of adverse drug reactions increases with age and with the number of drugs prescribed (Blazer, Federspiel, Ray, & Schaffner, 1983; Caranasos, Stewart, & Cluff, 1974; D'Arcy & McElnay, 1983; Gardner & Cluff, 1970; Greenblatt, Allen, & Shader, 1977; Hurwitz, 1969; Seidl, Thornton, Smith, & Cluff, 1966; Steel, Gertman, Crescenzi, & Anderson, 1981; Williamson & Chopin, 1980).

Adverse drug reactions afflict millions of people, cause hundreds of thousands of hospital admissions, result in thousands of deaths, and probably cost billions of dollars (Jick, 1974; U.S. Senate, 1976). In this country at least 3% of hospital admissions can be attributed to an adverse drug reaction (Caranasos, Stewart, & Cluff, 1974); in Great Britain, these reactions cause as many as 10% of admissions to geriatric beds (Williamson & Chopin, 1980).

Several factors contribute to the increased incidence of adverse drug reactions among the elderly. The pharmacology of many drugs changes with increasing age. Age-related alterations in both the pharmacokinetics and pharmacodynamics of potentially toxic drugs can result in adverse drug reactions. Details of these age-related changes in drug pharmacology are beyond the scope of this chapter; they are reviewed elsewhere in this book, as well as in several other texts and review articles (Conrad & Bressler, 1982; Jarvik, Greenblatt, & Harman, 1981; Kane, Ouslander, & Abrass, 1984; Lamy, 1980; Ouslander, 1981; Plein & Plein, 1981; Vestal, 1978).

Because elderly people are so finely balanced with their environment and have diminished homeostatic responses, they are especially susceptible to drug side effects (Kane et al., 1984). Side effects that may just be a nuisance to younger people—such as dry mouth, constipation, postural hypotension, and urinary frequency—may cause substantial disability in older people. Too often an adverse drug reaction disrupts the fine balance between the older person and the environment and precipitates delirium, dehydration, a fall, incontinence, or one of many other effects. These reactions are not only uncomfortable but can result in hospital admission, functional disability, other types of morbidity, and even death (Caranasos et al., 1974; D'Arcy & McElnay, 1983; Steel et al., 1981; Williamson & Chopin, 1980).

There is a myriad of potential adverse drug reactions in the elderly. Table 2.1 lists some of the more common ones; they are reviewed in detail elsewhere (D'Arcy & McElnay, 1983; Kane et al., 1984; Lamy, 1980). The frequency of specific adverse drug reactions depends upon the setting. In outpatient elderly populations, diuretics, digoxin antihypertensives, and psychotropic drugs are common causes of adverse drug reactions (Williamson & Chopin, 1980). In elderly patients in acute-care hospitals, vasodilators, antiarrhythmics, and other cardiovascular and psychotropic drugs are common offenders (Steel et al., 1981). Among elderly nursing home patients, psychotropic drugs cause numerous adverse reactions. There is considerable evidence that

TABLE 2.1
Examples of Common Adverse Drug Reactions in the Elderly

| Drug | Adverse Reactions |
|---|---|
| Diuretics | Dehydration, electrolyte imbalance, incontinence |
| Digoxin | Fatigue, anorexia, cardiac arrhythmias |
| Antihypertensives/vasodilators | Fatigue, mental status changes, hypotension, falls |
| Hypoglycemic agents | Hypoglycemia |
| Sedatives | Excessive sedation, other mental status changes |
| Antidepressants | Anticholinergic reactions,[a] cardiovascular problems,[b] sedation |
| Antipsychotics | Anticholinergic reactions, extrapyramidal reactions[c] |

[a]Dry mouth, blurry vision, constipation, tachycardia, urinary retention, reflux esophagitis, delirium
[b]Tricyclics; postural hypotension, delayed conduction, decreased myocardial contractility
[c]Bradykinesia, rigidity, tremor, dyskinesias, akathisia

this class of drugs is overprescribed and misused in this patient population (Ray et al., 1980; U.S. Senate, 1976). Their anticholinergic, cardiovascular, and central nervous system side effects can be especially problematic (see Table 2.1) (Blazer et al., Schaffner, 1983; Risch, Groom, & Janowsky, 1981; Thompson, Moran & Nies, 1983).

Polypharmacy increases the risk of adverse drug reactions not simply because of numbers but because the side effects of many commonly prescribed drugs in the elderly can be additive. Examples of this phenomenon include the combination of antihypertensives and psychotropic drugs, causing excessive sedation or hypotension, and the combination of tricyclic antidepressants and antiarrhythmics or beta blockers, causing decreased myocardial contractility.

## Drug–Drug Interactions

Polypharmacy obviously increases the risk of drug–drug interactions. There are literally hundreds of potential adverse drug interactions, and an extensive literature is available which reviews them in detail (Abramowicz, 1981; Armstrong, Driever, & Hays, 1980; Blaschke, Cohen, Tatro, & Rubin, 1981; D'Arcy, 1982, Roe, 1979).

Many of the drug–drug interactions described in the literature are of theoretical interest but hold little clinical significance. Clinically important drug–drug interactions are uncommon (Armstrong et al., 1980; Blaschke et al., 1981; Greenblatt, Abernethy, Morse, Harmatz, & Shader, 1984; Patriarca et al., 1983). For example, two reports (Bauman & Kimelblatt, 1982; Kramer & McClain, 1981) have suggested drug interactions that could be important in the elderly: the propensity of cimetidines to diminish the hepatic clearance of benzodiazepine drugs such as diazepam, and the depression of hepatic drug metabolism by influenza vaccine. More recent reports, however, have questioned the clinical significance of these interactions. Although cimetidine does increase the plasma concentration of diazepam and its active metabolite, central nervous system toxicity due to this interaction appears to be minimal (Greenblatt et al., 1984). This latter study, however, was done in a young subject population. In a study by Patriarca et al. (1983), no difference in incidence of toxicity of warfarin or theophylline was detected between nursing home patients who received influenza vaccine and those who did not.

Despite a lack of epidemiologic evidence, several types of drug–drug interactions could have clinical importance in the elderly (see Table 2.2). Drug–drug interactions can occur via a number of different mechanisms, ranging from alterations in drug absorption, distribution, metabolism, and excretion to pharmacologic antagonism or synergism between two or more agents. The potential for these types of interactions should always be considered when prescribing new drugs for an elderly patient.

## Drug–Patient Interactions

Probably of more clinical importance than drug–drug interactions in the elderly are what might be termed "drug–patient" interactions. This type of interaction implies an adverse drug reaction caused by the special sensitivity of an individual elderly

TABLE 2.2
Examples of Potentially Clinically Important Drug-Drug Interactions

| Type of Interaction | Examples | Clinical Implications |
|---|---|---|
| Interference with drug absorption | Antacids interacting with digoxin, INH antipsychotics | Diminished drug effectiveness |
| Displacement from binding proteins | Warfarin, oral hypo-glycemics, aspirin, chloral hydrate, other highly protein-bound drugs | Enhanced effects and increased risk of toxicity |
| Altered distribution | Digoxin and quinidine | Increased risk of toxicity |
| Altered metabolism | Cimetidine interacting with propranolol, theophylline, dilantin | Decreased drug clearance, enhanced effects, increased risk of toxicity |
| Altered excretion | Lithium and diuretics | Increased risk of toxicity and electrolyte imbalance |
| Pharmacological antagonism | Levodopa and clonidine | Decreased anti-parkinsonian effects |
| Pharmacological synergism | Tricyclic anti-depressants and antihypertensives | Increased risk of hypotension and mental status changes |

patient to a specific type of drug. Underlying chronic diseases and age-related biological and physiological changes make elderly people especially susceptible to these types of interactions. They are often less predictable than the effects of intrinsic liver and renal disease on drug pharmacology (Bennett et al., 1980; Williams, 1983).

Table 2.3 lists several examples of clinically important potential drug–patient interactions in the elderly. Several classes of drugs are especially hazardous in this regard. For example, beta blockers such as propranolol can block the sympathetic response to hypoglycemia in drug-treated diabetics, worsen hypoglycemia in diabetics as well as mask the symptoms, worsen bron-

**TABLE 2.3**
**Examples of Potentially Clinically Important Drug-Patient Interactions**

| Drug | Patient Factors | Clinical Implications |
|---|---|---|
| Diuretics | Diabetes | Decreased glucose tolerance |
|  | Poor nutritional status | Increased risk of dehydration and electrolyte imbalance |
| Beta blockers | Diabetes | Sympathetic response to hypoglycemia masked |
|  | Chronic obstructive lung disease | Increased bronchospasm |
|  | Congestive heart failure | Decreased myocardial contractility |
|  | Peripheral vascular disease | Increased claudication |
| Tricyclic antidepressants | Congestive heart failure, angina | Tachycardia, decreased myocardial contractility, postural hypotension exacerbating cardiovascular conditions |
| Tricyclic antidepressants, antihistamines, and other drugs with anticholinergic effects | Constipation, glaucoma and other visual impairments, prostatic hyperplasia, reflux esophagitis | Worsening of symptoms |
| Antipsychotics | Parkinsonism | Worsening of immobility |
| Psychotropics | Dementia | Further impairment of cognitive function |

chospasm in patients with obstructive lung disease, exacerbate congestive heart failure, and increase symptomatic peripheral vascular disease. Drugs with anticholinergic effects (of which there are many) can worsen chronic symptoms such as constipation, urinary hesitancy, and reflux esophagitis and can precipitate glaucoma, fecal impaction, and urinary retention in susceptible elderly patients. Many conditions that are subclinical in elderly patients, such as mild congestive heart failure and prostatic hyperplasia, may become clinically manifest as the result of drug treatment.

Thus, when prescribing a new drug for an elderly patient, the possibility should always be considered that the patient, because of an underlying condition, may be especially susceptible to the side effects of certain types of drugs.

## Poor Compliance

Polypharmacy is among the many factors that contribute to poor compliance with drug regimens in the elderly population. The incidence of noncompliance is disturbingly high, even in young people treated with a single drug (Haynes, Taylor, & Sackett, 1979). It is well known that about half of the people who are prescribed drugs do not adhere properly to a drug regimen (Haynes et al., 1979). Surveys of elderly people suggest poor compliance is even more common with increasing age (Gryfe & Gryfe, 1984; Lundin, 1978; Schwartz, Wang, Zeitz, & Goss, 1962). The prescription of multiple drugs in complicated dosing regimens certainly exacerbates the problem of noncompliance. Without some type of aid such as a specially designed container or charting system, it is highly unlikely that elderly people will take three or more drugs, some once a day, some three or four times a day, some before meals, some after meals, and so forth. When added to other barriers to compliance, which include socioeconomic, cultural, physical, and psychological factors (Haynes et al., 1979; Ouslander, 1981; Schwartz, Wang, Zeita, & Goss, 1962), complex drug regimens may serve as the final blow to an elderly person's ability to comply with drug therapy.

## Increased Costs

Polypharmacy results in increased costs to patients, institutions, and the public in general. Many elderly people live on a fixed and limited income. Because outpatient drug prescriptions are not covered under Medicare, elderly people may spend a substantial amount of money on drugs. Minimizing the number of drugs and the duration of drug therapy, especially some of the newer, more expensive preparations, will help elderly people to manage their overall health care expenditures better.

Both acute-care hospitals and nursing homes can have increased costs because of polypharmacy. Medicare's recent initiation of prospective reimbursement for hospitals will impose new financial constraints on these institutions. The costs of the pharmacy are likely to be examined more closely. Polypharmacy not only increases costs because of the costs of drugs themselves; more drugs and drug doses result in greater amounts of pharmacy and nursing staff time in preparing and administering the medications. These considerations also apply to nursing homes, where a substantial amount of nursing time is spent preparing and administering drugs. Because close to half of all nursing home care is funded by Medicaid through fixed daily rates, reduction in nursing time for dealing with drugs could result in savings to the nursing home or, more important, more staff time for the personal, social, and rehabilitative aspects of nursing home care.

Ultimately the costs of polypharmacy—the drugs themselves, the hospital and nursing home staff time, and the care of patients who suffer adverse drug reactions—is borne by all of us because a substantial proportion of the costs of health care for the elderly are covered by Medicare and Medicaid.

## WHAT CAN BE DONE ABOUT POLYPHARMACY?

There is a clear need to educate health professionals as well as the public about the hazards of polypharmacy. Didactic material about geriatric pharmacology should be incorporated into all medical-school curricula, medical and pharmacology textbooks, and continuing education programs. A recent study indicated that a more personal approach to physicians, using educational visits by clinical pharmacists and a series of mailed "unadvertisements," substantially reduced the incidence of prescription and the costs of several drugs (Avorn & Soumerai, 1983). Clinical pharmacists can be helpful in acute-care hospital and nursing home settings by carefully reviewing drug regimens and discussing optimal pharmacologic management with physicians and nurses. Many states actually require consultant pharmacists to review drug utilization in nursing homes. Also, computer programs have been developed that can detect potential drug interactions (Armstrong et al., 1980; Blaschke et al., 1981). Local quality assurance and utilization review committees can serve to reinforce efforts to minimize polypharmacy and its attendant hazards.

Educational efforts also should be directed at the elderly population. Elderly people should understand the potential problems that can result from polypharmacy and should be encouraged to seek appropriate information from their physician or other health professionals (such as a pharmacist) about each drug they have been prescribed. Patients should be encouraged to question the need for starting or continuing a medication, and they should be discouraged as much as possible from seeking a drug as the solution to their health problem. In addition, patients should carry with them an updated record of the drugs they take and should bring their pill bottles with them to office or clinic visits. Information pamphlets can serve as useful vehicles for transmitting this information to the elderly population. They can be produced rather inexpensively by medical centers and local agencies involved in health care for the elderly, or through small foundation grants, and they can be distributed in hospitals, clinics, physicians' offices, pharmacies, and senior centers.

The problem of polypharmacy will persist, however, until physicians alter their prescribing habits. The following are several basic principles for prescribing drugs for the elderly (Ouslander, 1981; Vestal, 1978):

1. Prescribing drug treatment only when absolutely necessary.
2. Avoiding interactions between newly prescribed drugs, drugs already being taken, and underlying conditions in a given elderly patient.
3. Minimizing drug doses and simplifying dosing regimens as much as possible.

4. Carefully monitoring patients for compliance, drug effects, and symptoms or signs of adverse drug reactions.
5. Discontinuing drug treatment as soon as medically possible.

Only through adherence to these principles will polypharmacy and its hazards be minimized.

# 3

# Pharmacology and the Elderly in Social Perspective

*Bess Dana*
*Michael N. Mulvilhill*

In recent years, scientific investigations of both a laboratory and clinical nature have been increasingly successful in illuminating the biomedical pathways that link pharmacology with the aging process. At the same time, the growing incidence and prevalence of drug misuse, abuse, and nonuse among the elderly strongly suggests that too much of the gain in biomedical understanding of the pharmacology-aging relationship is lost in its translation into the actual medical care of the elderly patient.

Elderly patients, for instance, represent a disproportionate number of the patients subject to adverse drug reactions during the course of their hospital stay. They are more likely than younger patients to be admitted to the hospital because of drug-related symptoms. Although they account for the greatest expenditures for prescription drugs, the elderly also are associated with the highest rate of noncompliance with drug regimens (Caranasos et al., 1974; Gomolin & Chapron, 1983). Even though present epidemiological investigations are confined to the population of the elderly receiving medical care rather than to the elderly population at large, a wide discrepancy clearly exists between the optimism of the biomedical message and the pessimism of current epidemiological findings.

The sense of hope conveyed by the biomedical message is further diminished by the consistent epidemiological finding that increased risk for adverse outcomes from drug treatment is associated with advancing age (Lamy, 1983). In light of the changing demography of aging—which already shows an increased growth in the number of elderly persons 85 years of age and over and projects an acceleration of this growth pattern in the years ahead—the present discrepancy between the therapeutic possibilities of modern pharmacology and the actual outcomes of drug treatment can be expected to grow in direct proportion to the increase in the number of the old-old in the elderly population.

This chapter examines the conditions of the social, psychological, and health care environment for clues to understanding and dealing with the troubled and troubling relationship between modern pharmacology and the elderly. In pursuit of this general purpose, we will (1) place the relationship between drugs and the elderly within a social-behavioral frame of reference; (2) identify those particular factors in the social, psychological, and health care delivery environment that influence this relationship; (3) establish a linkage between the generic and specific components that are implicated in the drugs-and-the-elderly problem and its solution; and (4) recommend next steps for preventive and remedial action in education, research, social health policy and planning, and the delivery of social health services.

# SOCIAL AND BEHAVIORAL INFLUENCES ON THE RELATIONSHIP BETWEEN DRUGS AND THE ELDERLY

Throughout the developmental history of modern medicine, numerous wide-ranging and interrelated personal and social factors have been identified as obstacles to the effective application of advances in biomedical knowledge to the health care of the individual patient at any phase in the life cycle. The gap that currently exists between the biomedical possibilities for improving the health status of the elderly patient through age-conscious drug therapy and the probability of the patient's actually benefitting from such treatment represents a striking example of the uneasy relationship that still exists between the elements of medical science, medical care, and the personal and social environment. While neither the problems of drug use and abuse nor their social and behavioral connotations are unique to the aging population, the lack of fit between the demands of most drug regimens for self-management and the physical, psychological, and social changes associated with advancing age warrants the definition of the problem in specific as well as generic terms.

A growing number of studies that attempt such problem definition are beginning to appear in the gerontological literature. Despite this numerical growth, the reported studies still lag far behind age-related biomedical investigations in quantity, scope, and methodological sophistication. The inferences that can be drawn from their findings, however, are too consistent to be dismissed because of such common failings as small sample size and selection bias, the lack of controls, their retrospective rather than prospective derivation, and their descriptive rather than analytic nature. Even if not definitive, they certainly identify specific areas that warrant further inquiry and provide useful clues for changes that can be safely introduced into traditional health care practice without further validation.

The doctor, the patient, and the relationship between them occupy a prominent place in the studies, case reports, essays, and editorial comments that comprise the literature reviewed. The prototypical prescribing behavior of the physician that emerges from these sources is characterized by (1) the use of the same criteria established for younger and healthier patients in determining the drug regimen for the elderly patient; (2) the failure to take into account, in renewing a prescription or ordering new medication, other prescription as well as over-the-counter drugs and nutrients that the elderly patient may be taking; (3) inadequate explanation of the "rules" for drug usage, including when, how, and for how long a particular medication should be taken; (4) the neglect of the responsibility to alert the patient to possible side effects of the prescribed medication and/or to provide instructions as to what to do in the event of an adverse drug reaction; and (5) the tendency to let personal feelings about aging itself interfere with the exercise of objective clinical judgment in deciding whether, how, and if to treat (Fedder, 1982; Lamy, 1983).

The prototypical drug-taking behavior of the elderly patient, as described in the literature, appears to be no less problem ridden than the prescribing behavior of the physician. The high incidence of noncompliance; multiple drug usage, including over-the-counter as well as prescription drugs; and the failure to understand the proper timing and dosages of medications are commonly cited as evidence of the elderly patient's poor accommodation to the demands of drug management. The literature affirms that the very physical and psychological deficits that drug therapy is designed to alleviate frequently militate against the elderly patient's capacity to assume the personal responsibilities upon which the achievement of optimum therapeutic benefits depends. However, the much-needed data that indicate how the elderly actually reconcile the daily tasks of drug management with the resources and routines of daily living are just beginning to be reported.

Brody and her colleagues at the Philadelphia Geriatric Center (Brody, Kleban, & Moles, 1983) have led the way in developing a methodology and generating findings that show us how older persons' perceptions of their symptoms, general system of health beliefs, and personal health practices influence the way they function in their role as personal health care managers. By moving the locus of inquiry from the house of medicine to the elderly person's home and community, the investigators have been able (1) to capture facets of the drug-taking behavior of older people that are rarely observed or elicited in the intimidating environment of the clinical encounter, and (2) to demonstrate the linkages between the elderly's self-assessment of their symptoms on a day-to-day basis, their health beliefs and practices, and their use or misuse of drugs.

Brody cautions against the temptation to generalize the findings from a small, nonrepresentative urban sample of the elderly to the health behavior of the elderly population at large. It is not necessary to overstretch the data, however, in order to point out the insights to be derived from directing the search for explanations of older persons' drug-taking behavior toward better understanding of their own attitudes toward and subjective perceptions of their illness, the place of illness in their own personal scheme of things, and the social and fiscal costs versus benefits to be derived from adherence to a drug regimen.

In their review of the literature pertaining to the sociobehavioral determinants of compliance, Becker et al. (1977) point out that earlier investigations of the social and behavioral components of the relationship between drugs and the elderly have been helpful in identifying the "quantifiable characteristics of the patient (e.g., demographic and social), the regimen (e.g., type, complexity, discomfort, duration), and the illness (e.g., medically defined seriousness, duration, disability)" (Becker et al., 1977, p. 40). They indicate, however, that this use of a medical model to explain patient behavior "has the advantage of measurement, but the disadvantage that one does not always understand well the meaning of such associations" (p. 41). The health belief model that Brody and her colleagues employ begins to correct for the limitation of vision resulting from the exclusive reliance on a medical model to explain personal and social behavior.

The findings from the Philadelphia Geriatric Center's community-based research, coupled with the recently published results from a study of the medication behavior of 183 elderly apartment residents conducted by members of the Department of Pharmaceutics, School of Pharmacy, University of Washington (Hammarlund, Ostrom, & Kethley, 1985), strongly suggest that the disturbing statistical evidence of noncompliance and adverse drug reactions among the elderly expresses the social and psychological as well as biological vulnerability of older persons to medical interventions designed to counteract and/or contain the adverse physical and mental changes associated with aging.

Such seemingly simple tasks as opening "childproof" bottles

can present a major obstacle to the older person with arthritic hands; reading the fine print on a drug label may be an impossibility for the visually impaired older person; and, to the older person suffering from memory loss, the differing time schedules and dosages of the multiple drugs that are likely to appear on the medication menu of the elderly may not only be difficult to understand but lead to unintentional violations with serious physical consequences (Comfort, 1983). These instrumental problems are compounded by the feelings that "nobody cares," "nothing can be done," and "I don't want to bother anyone," which have been reported by both the Philadelphia and Seattle studies as characteristic of their respective elderly study samples. It becomes easy to see how social isolation, low self-esteem, and apathy emerge as poignant and powerful risk factors for negative therapeutic outcomes of drug treatment.

Despite differences in the conceptual models that guide the search for social and behavioral clues to the problems associated with drug treatment of the elderly, investigators concur in the importance they ascribe to the doctor-patient transaction as the vehicle for helping the elderly patient to understand and make appropriate use of drug therapy in the management of his or her health problems. Particular reliance is placed on the power of educational strategies to bring about changes in physicians' prescribing behavior, changes that incorporate knowledge and understanding of the biology, psychology, and sociology of aging in (1) obtaining a drug history from the patient, (2) selecting an age-adjusted drug regimen for the patient, (3) helping the older patient understand the importance of the prescribed medication(s), and (4) providing clear instructions and ongoing support to the patient in fulfilling his or her responsibilities in the management of drug therapy. The underlying assumption in most of the educational approaches described is that, given the proper learning opportunities for broadening and deepening their knowledge and sensitivity to the special needs of the elderly patient, physicians will be able to establish and maintain a partnership relationship with their patients in the achievement of optimum benefits from the prescribed therapeutic regimen.

# SOCIAL POLICY AND SOCIAL SYSTEM VARIABLES: THE MISSING ELEMENTS

Absent from the preceding formulation of both the problem of drug use and misuse among the elderly and the proposed solutions is more than passing reference to the influence of social policy and social system variables on the behavior of both physicians and older persons and on the nature of the relationship between them. Yet, the major advances that have been made in addressing the health needs of the aging have come about through continuing efforts to establish and maintain a circular relationship between and among social policy; the organization, delivery, and financing of health and health-related services; and the personal health care of the individual older person. Seen from this perspective, the relationship between drugs and the elderly, if it is to be fully understood in social and behavioral terms, must be considered as part of rather than apart from the overall health care of the individual older patient. It is thus subject to the same conditions of the medical and social environment that exert an increasingly powerful influence on the scope, substance, and style of personal health services for all Americans, regardless of age. What is currently identified as "wrong" with this relationship as reflected in physician and patient behavior may in fact be a measure of what is "wrong" with the scope, organization, delivery style, and financing of health and health-related services as they relate to the particular needs and wants of the aging population. Based on this premise, the process of righting these wrongs may well necessitate changing policy and system behavior as a condition for bringing about change in the behavior of the physician, the older patient, and the relationship between them.

The degree to which such common manifestations of this problem as noncompliance, adverse drug reactions, or under- or overprescribing of medications serve as metaphors for disorders in the social health system has, as yet, not been scientifically assessed or validated. Inferences can be drawn, however, from the findings of small-scale pilot studies, demonstration projects, and the emerging literature pertaining to the impact of new policies and regulatory practices on health and social services to the aging. These inferences support the assumption that such behavioral attributes of the health care system as accessibility, continuity, and outreach to and coordination with family and community-based support systems are implicated in the older person's capacity to make optimum use of medical recommendations.

For example, Haynes and Sackett (1976), in their comprehensive review of studies of the determinants of patients' compliance, point out that, when analysis of the complex subject of the patient-therapist interaction as it affects compliance is

> restricted to those features of the patient-therapist interaction for which data are both sufficient and of a consistent nature, two clear features emerge. First, all studies of the relationship between the degree of supervision and compliance found positive associations. Thus hospitalized patients are more compliant than day-patients, who in turn are more compliant than out-patients. Furthermore, that this link is causal has been strongly supported by pre and post studies showing improvement in compliance when the frequency of out-patient visits is increased, when home visits are added, when the patient's family is recruited in supervision, when objective evidence of noncompliance is fed back to the patient, and when greater continuity of care is provided. [Haynes & Sackett, 1976, p. 35]

Beyond the success reported in changing patient behavior through the modification of system behavior, the strategies reported by Haynes and Sackett (1976) and replicated or applied in the design and implementation of other small-scale and usually short-term studies or demonstration projects support both the need for and value of expanding the scope of research and demonstration projects to include the design and assessment of creative ways of modifying the organization and deployment of human and material resources to support, supplement, and/or enhance patients' and/or physicians' capacities to meet their respective responsibilities in the management of health problems.

The health decision model for understanding and improving patient compliance developed by Eraker, Kirscht, and Becker (1984) represents an important effort in this direction. Their proposed model is designed to help physicians overcome what they describe as their "conceptual difficulty of fitting the potential components of needed interventions into an organized program [to improve cooperation with treatment]" (p. 260). It relates compliance interventions to "modifying the therapeutic recommendations to reflect patient preferences, modifying current experiences, enhancing knowledge, and modifying social interaction factors" (p. 260).

A variety of strategies based on the findings of earlier studies of compliance are recommended as ways of translating the model into the daily acts of patient care. These include (1) modifying the therapeutic regimen to accommodate to patient preference; (2) establishing a contingency contract, wherein both parties set forth a treatment goal, the specific obligations of each party in attempting to accomplish that goal, and a time for its achievement; (3) involving other personnel (e.g., nurses and pharmacists) in the provision of instruction, clarification, and reinforcement; (4) modifying social interaction factors such as social networks, and (5) extending supervision beyond the patient's stay at the office or health facility, "through reminder telephone calls, home visits, [and] instructing the patient to keep a record of which pills were taken each day and at what times" (Eraker et al., 1984, pp. 261–262).

The collaborative work of Eraker et al. (1984) makes clear that, inside the medical model, which until recently has dominated the definition and solution of health problems, is a social health model struggling to emerge. The health decision model that they propose shortens the distance that separates medical from social interventions. Still missing from their careful delineation of the elements that constitute a new blueprint for dealing with the problems of noncompliance is the consideration of the influence of organizational characteristics, payment mechanisms, eligibility requirements, and social provisions regarding the capacity of both providers and consumers of health and social services to meet their respective responsibilities as implicated in the health decision model. Eraker et al. do point out the deficiencies of medical educators in teaching their students (1) to recognize the conditions under which the patient can be expected to follow advice and (2) to develop "the interview skills needed to assess what the patient knows, believes, or is concerned about" (p. 264). The authors fail, however, to call attention to such deficiencies in the medical care delivery system as the imbalance between the quality and quantity of hospital and ambulatory care services, the fragmentation and discontinuity of care, and the acute-disease focus of admitting policies and diagnostic and treatment practices that militate against the translation of the health decision model into consumer-oriented personal care services.

## POLICY, REGULATIONS, AND THE RELATIONSHIP BETWEEN DRUGS AND THE ELDERLY

There has been much anxiety created for both health care providers and consumers by the increasingly vocal presence of government in the conduct of the daily acts of patient care, as symbolized by TEFRA (the Tax Equity and Fiscal Responsibility Act of 1982) and its regulatory expression in the DRG (diagnosis-related group) reimbursement formula for the hospital care of Medicare recipients. Ironically enough, this anxiety has been more effective than the literature in setting in motion or accelerating a much-needed reexamination of the behavioral characteristics of the health care system as they relate to the changing demography, health care problems, and personal and social resources of the population served. Even at this early stage in the activation of the DRG program as a fact of hospital life, the very process of compliance with the mandate to contain the length of hospital stay appears to some observers to have heightened the attending physician's awareness of the need for continuing institutionally or community-based "step-down" health and social services as a means for maintaining continuity of medical care and helping the patient meet the responsibilities of daily living. In recognition of this need, many acute-care hospitals are themselves developing long-term care services; others are expanding the traditional discharge planning function to include case management as a means of "affording physicians and thus their patients access to health and social services as they exist in the community" (Brody & Magel, 1984, pp. 627–628).

Few older patients leave the hospital without at least one drug prescription in hand; the older the patient, the greater the number of prescriptions is likely to be; and, given the multiple illnesses associated with advancing age and the specialty orientation of modern medicine, the greater the likelihood that polypharmacy and polyphysiciancy will march hand in hand. What the patient is far less likely to have is a social prescription that (1) recognizes the relationship between the recommended drug regimen and the patient's capacities for its management and (2) facilitates access to the resources needed to support or supplement these capacities. The increased attention to the development and implementation of systematic approaches to the provision of "short-term long-term" (Brody & Magel, 1984, p. 678) health and social services holds promise for preventing an increase in the incidence of drug reactions that, without continuing medical supervision and support services, may well result from shortened hospital stays.

While the implications of shorter hospital stays on the health status of the elderly receives continued coverage in both the public and professional press, comparatively little attention has been paid to the other side of the TEFRA coin: the impact that DRG-related changes in hospital admitting policies and practices may have on the elderly patient's access to hospital services. Nor have the possible limitations in access imposed by the increase in the cost-sharing formula mandated by recent changes in Medicare regulations aroused the public and professional concern that they would seem to warrant.

The issue of access as it affects older persons' utilization of health services in general and their drug utilization behavior in particular has been insufficiently investigated to warrant the persistent assumption in the literature that Medicare has solved the access problem. The fact that most of what is known about the elderly's utilization characteristics is derived from studies of patients already under medical care may have contributed to the virtual disappearance of the access issue from the vocabulary of health services research. Whether it also has disappeared from the vocabulary of the elderly remains a question that warrants renewed investigation.


## FROM REACTION TO ACTION: A LOOK AT THE FUTURE

Given the fickle nature of many of the social and economic policies and regulatory changes through which the federal government's concept of social responsibility has been expressed in the first half of the 1980s, predictions of the ultimate impact of the recent changes in fiscal policy and practices on consumer, provider, or systems behavior come very close to being speculation. It would seem more productive to focus our attention on what needs to be done to enable consumers and providers to become the leaders rather than the followers in adapting policy, systems, and professional behavior to the needs of the population served. In turning from reaction to action as the appropriate behavioral stance of the health and social service community, high priority should be given to changing the current governmental commitment to reducing the fiscal costs of health and health-related services to a commitment to reducing the social costs of illness and its care.

The current status of the relationship between drugs and the elderly indicates measures are needed to reduce the mounting social costs of illness and disability among the aging. The following need to be addressed:

1. Broadening the scope of inquiry into the health behavior of the elderly to include the population of the elderly as a whole, through the design and implementation of community-based as well as institutionally based research and demonstration projects.
2. Acknowledging the interdisciplinary and interinstitutional nature of so-called "health needs and problems" in policy making, planning, and service delivery.
3. Including interprofessional community-based opportunities as an integral part of educational programs designed to

enhance the capacity of the future social worker, nurse, physician, and health manager to make optimum use of finite human material resources in addressing the social costs of health problems of the elderly.

Values as well as knowledge are deeply implicated in the changes involved in the designing and implementing of a social health model for the appropriate expression of professional responsiveness to the needs and rights of the aging. The unifying requirement for all of us is, above all, the willingness to put social needs and goals, whether individually, institutionally, or universally expressed, ahead of professional self-interests in the definition and implementation of our tasks and responsibilities.

# Part II
# Issues in Nutrition

# Introduction

Studies of nutrition and aging encompass not only the biological and medical sciences but also sociocultural, economic, and behavioral aspects of food and eating. The authors of chapters in this section agree that the elderly are at nutritional risk because they are vulnerable to diseases, affected by public policy discussions about income support and medical care, and susceptible to simple solutions to complex problems. These multifaceted vulnerabilities require the application of knowledge from a variety of disciplines, and there is no doubt that much work is needed to address the issues of nutrition and the elderly.

Watkin (Chapter 4) considers aging after maturity to be a disease that requires a scientific model for investigating prolonged survival. He believes that nutrition as prevention and treatment of aging has too long been a "political football" for those in the field of social advocacy, and that it must be restored to experienced professionals to provide genuine assistance for the improvement of the health of millions of Americans. He states that nutrition as therapy requires the provision of sufficient energy in the diet, especially fat and carbohydrates, to overcome the primary nutrient deficiency among the elderly. This is certainly true for many elderly persons; however, it also must be recognized that energy requirements are generally much lower, due to decreased body cell mass and reduced levels of activity. Diets, therefore, must be nutrient-dense, since all other nutrient requirements remain the same or may even be increased. Dr. Watkin emphasizes the importance of sufficient protein and encourages increased calcium intake for everyone throughout life. He concludes by supporting the continuation of public food and income programs now in place and urges the combining of resources in gerontology, medicine, and nutrition in order to increase survival.

Spencer and colleagues (Chapter 5) discuss the issue of calcium in greater detail. Spencer has devoted much of her research career to the study of osteoporosis, a major public health problem. This disease is most often discovered after a debilitating skeletal fracture has occurred, when, even if diagnosed earlier, the process is already much advanced. Spencer et al. emphasize the lifelong importance of adequate calcium intake, particularly in females, and present data from Spencer's research that indicate that the long-held views of adaptation to low calcium intake, resulting in concomitant calcium adequacy, are not correct. Indeed, her studies appear to confirm other investigators' results that recommend increasing calcium intake for optimal bone mass from the current Recommended Dietary Allowance (RDA) of 800 mg/day to 1500 mg/day. However, they caution that there still is no scientific proof for the calcium-related etiology of osteoporosis. Spencer, Kramer, and Osis discuss the effects of phosphorus and protein on calcium absorption and conclude by describing the interactions of aluminum-containing antacids and alcohol on bone loss and osteoporosis.

Social, cultural, and economic issues in nutrition are reviewed by Kart (Chapter 6). From his perspective as a sociologist, he emphasizes the problems the elderly poor have in obtaining, preparing, and enjoying food. He supports the establishment of a strong national nutrition policy, one that would expand the present food and income maintenance programs. He chides nutrition experts for failing to achieve consensus on these issues. Kart uses the court case of Mary Hier, a 92-year-old psychiatric hospital resident with feeding and drug administration problems, to demonstrate that provision of food is a medical treatment. Kart views the court's decision about her continuing care as neglecting the sentiment and symbolism of food and feeding in our society. His compassionate approach to the poor and lonely elderly might serve to remind policy makers that more than dollars and science are required to assure provision of sufficient food.

Promises of simple cures are especially attractive to the elderly. Hershey (Chapter 7) presents several interesting and even amusing examples of food fads and diet remedies. Whether based on erroneous scientific reasoning or untested theories, the appeal may seem reasonable to the poorly informed or desperate elderly person. While some of these remedies may do no harm to those who are healthy and well nourished, they may be very expensive for those who can least afford them. For those who suffer from chronic diseases or malnutrition, dietary imbalances created by some of these regimens may indeed cause harm or may replace proven, reliable therapies. The elderly also are vulnerable to drug fads, some of which produce adverse effects and in addition are not likely to be reimbursed by medical insurance. Hershey advocates public information as the best hope against the continuing dissemination of misinformation.

G.J.P.

# 4

# The Disease: Aging;
# The Therapy: Nutrition

*Donald M. Watkin*

## THE DISEASE

Aging after maturity is a disease that is inexorable, ubiquitous, and varies among members of the human species only by the rapidity with which it occurs. A comparison of the survival curve of ancient Rome with that of today shows that great strides in postponing death have been made during the last 2,000 years (see Figure 4.1). Much of that progress occurred in the past century, an example of the time implosion. Reductions in infant and maternal mortality, child mortality, famine, and pestilence and the introduction of safe water and food supplies and hygienic methods of waste disposal, together with more recent biochemical approaches to the control of infectious and neoplastic disease, have created what some have described as "rectangularization" of the survival curve, or the compression of morbidity (Fries, 1984).

Relatively little progress has been made in the 2,000 years since ancient Rome in increasing the technical lifespan of humans (TLS$^h$), the oldest documented age to which a human being is known to have survived. The current record of 120 years was achieved by a Japanese man (McWhirter, 1983), thus providing a basis for using 120 as the TLS$^h$. History and modern molecular biology strongly suggest that aging is genetically

61

FIGURE 4.1    Survival-Rate Improvement, Ancient Rome versus 1984 versus 2084

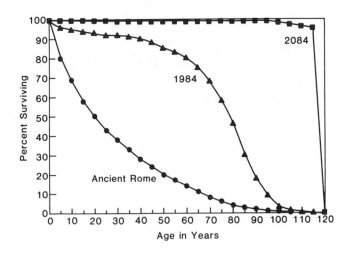

programmed, with death scheduled for all humans at no later than about 120 years of age. This in turn suggests that a reasonable goal for modern medicine is to rectangularize survival by approaching premature death as a disease preventable by application of the same philosophy and methods that have reduced to insignificance other diseases that once exacted so terrible a toll from society.

Unfortunately, survival for most humans fails to approximate the TLS[h]. As shown in Figure 4.2, the log of the death rate begins to rise linearly at age 30, with a doubling rate of about 8 years through age 80. Recently, more accurate data have become available on the age at death of persons up to 80 years old. Figure 4.3 shows that the doubling rate among these older persons is slowed from 8 to approximately 14 years. This suggests that persons with the genetic constitution for survival are increasing in number, in part at least because they have not died earlier from diseases now preventable by public health measures and treatable by modern medicine. This contributes to the rapid increase in numbers of very old persons, which poses formidable problems that have been anticipated by scientists for years and are now receiving the attention of the mass media (Centenarians, 1984; Otten, 1984).

Studies of persons in this age group are few. One of the best, now being conducted at the University of Kentucky in Lexington (Thompson et al., 1984), has found distributions of human lymphocyte antigens (HLA's) in centenarians to be different from those encountered in younger populations. They also have found these centenarians to have a reversal of the ratio of helper/inducer to suppressor/killer T-lymphocytes that has been reported in younger persons with protein-energy malnutrition (Chandra, 1983). This latter finding poses the question of whether this deterioration of cellular immunity is programmed in genes or is a direct result of inadequate intake of energy and protein during late maturity.

This question illustrates the need to approach aging as a disease and to investigate it using the scientific medical model. If the investigators in Kentucky find the problem is nutritional, the cellular immune deficiencies may be treated in the centenarians and prevented in those who are younger by appropriate attention to nutritional intervention.

**FIGURE 4.2   Gompertz Plot, Age 20 through Age 84**

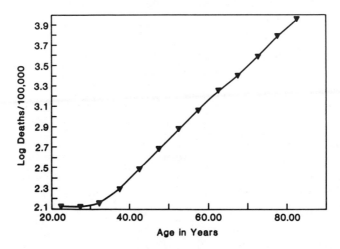

*Source*: National Center for Health Statistics, Washington, D.C., May 25, 1984.

FIGURE 4.3    Gompertz Plot, Age 20 through Age 120

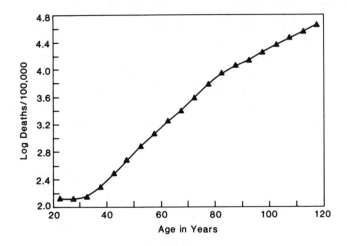

*Source*: National Center for Health Statistics, Washington, D.C., May 25, 1984.

Using the scientific medical model, society has eradicated sources of disease and accidents that took the lives of many persons who could have survived to 100 or more. When society seriously looks upon aging as a disease and not solely a social problem, progress truly will be made toward the goal of rectangularizing the survival curve.

Nutrition, a universal prerequisite of life, is an ideal focus for study because of its role as the primary therapeutic agent in the prevention and treatment of virtually every cause of disability known to humankind. Universal and foremost among those causes of disability is the disease aging. Nutrition has not yet been applied to the prevention and treatment of aging because aging has become a political football.

In its initial conceptualization as Title VII of the Older Americans Act of 1965, as amended, the Nutrition Program for Older Americans (NPOA) was conceived as the ideal vehicle for delivering global support to older Americans. Complications in the legislative process delayed its implementation for 18 months (Watkin, 1983) and enabled the then-named and fully-funded Title III program to become entrenched. As a result, when

NPOA did become a well-funded institution, its resources were coveted by the so-called Area Agency on Aging community. Nonetheless, with firm congressional backing, NPOA, now named Title III$_c$, has continued to be the most popular feature of the Older Americans Act of 1965, as amended. This is primarily because nutrition encompasses every aspect of life. Nutrition is the magnet attracting older Americans to locations, facilities, and persons who can assist them in resolving virtually every problem posed by human existence.

In industry and government, one of the buzzwords of the 1980s has been the Employee Assistance Program (EAP). The EAP, in a given environment, is meant to provide assistance in resolving problems of (1) substance abuse, including alcohol abuse; (2) marriage; (3) law; (4) finance; and (5) mental and physical health, as well as difficulties with poor performance on the job. Most employers feel that they gain back at least $5 for every $1 invested in the program. NPOA affords an equal opportunity to the elderly and aged persons of this nation.

In an even broader context, nutrition is the route to prevention of a very broad spectrum of maladies over the entire life cycle of the human population. In alphabetical order, nutrition is concerned with arthritis, cachexia, cancer, cardiovascular disease, dermatology, dentistry, diabetology, endocrinology, infectious diseases, intelligence, neurology, obesity, osteopenia, psychiatry, and the special senses, to mention just a few. Furthermore, nutrition is benign, unthreatening, and offers the appeal of the good qualities associated with God, mother, the home, and apple pie. It involves agriculture, animal husbandry, transportation, food processing, packaging, merchandising, advertising, distribution, marketing, consumer affairs, and even Wall Street. In politics, it stands its ground in both the U.S. Senate and the U.S. House of Representatives against any competing issue.

These qualities have led many faddists and quacks to seize it as a means of laughing all the way to the bank. It is time for nutrition to be restored to those who have the professional expertise to provide genuine assistance to the millions of Americans who are now victims of chicanery. This can be done by using nutrition as the prime vehicle for improving health; increasing effective longevity; and controlling, until very close to the TLS[h], the ravages of the disease of aging.

The scope of nutrition is immense. It is the vehicle for providing health education to all ages, from children through the aged. Through the expansion of nutrition programs and other nutrition-related resources already in being, persons of all ages will learn what is required to stay alive long enough to closely approach the TLS[h].

## NUTRITION AS HEALTH PROMOTION

Reports of a series of studies in California (Belloc, 1973; Belloc & Breslow, 1972; Belloc, Breslow, & Hochstim, 1971) dramatically demonstrate the value of health promotion and indicate clearly the crucial role nutrition plays in such promotion. The authors devised a parameter called a "RIDIT," an acronym for the expression "Relative to an Identified Distribution." A RIDIT approaching zero suggests good health, a lack of complaints, and a high level of energy. As the RIDIT approaches unity, disability is grave and the prognosis ominous.

The California investigators next related the RIDIT values found in the study population to the degree to which these same people adhered to seven health practices. These practices are (1) eat a balanced diet, (2) eat on a regular schedule, (3) avoid tobacco, (4) avoid alcohol abuse, (5) engage in regularly scheduled physical activity, (6) obtain the required amount of sleep daily, and (7) enjoy regularly scheduled rest and relaxation. Some people did not follow any of these practices; some only a few; and some followed all seven. As shown in Figure 4.4, the greater the number of health practices followed throughout life, the lower (and hence better) the average physical health RIDIT, by age group. The elderly persons of 80 who had followed all seven health practices had the same RIDITS as the 35 year olds who had followed from zero to two. These findings confirm the effectiveness and cost effectiveness of health promotion. Since at least five of the seven health practices are nutrition related, they also indicate the value of the incorporation of nutrition into global schemes for health promotion.

FIGURE 4.4   Average RIDIT According to Number of Health Practices
Followed, by Age Group

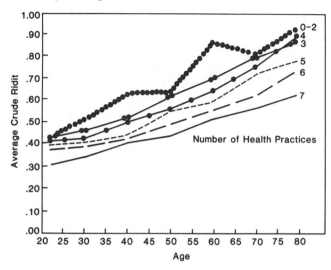

*Source*: N. B. Belloc and L. Breslow. (1972). Relationship of physical health status and
health practices. *Preventive Medicine, 1*, 409–421, Figure 1. Used by permission.

## NUTRITION AS THERAPY

Before detailing the accomplishments of applying the knowledge we have of nutrition, let us define the terms *elderly* and
*aged*. *Elderly* persons are those aged 80 through 89; *aged* are
those aged 90 or over (Watkin, 1984).

### Energy

The primary nutrient deficiency among the elderly and the
aged is energy (Abraham, Carroll, Dresser, & Johnson, 1977b;
Schaefer, 1982). Failure to consume enough energy reduces the
ability to expend energy, as was clearly demonstrated throughout occupied Europe during World War II and in the re-
nowned Minnesota studies of human starvation (Keys, Brozek,
Henschel, Mickelsen, & Taylor, 1950). Andres (1981) has suggested that relative overweight, about 115 percent of "ideal"

defined by the 1959 Metropolitan Life Insurance recommendations (Metropolitan Life Insurance Company, 1959), affords
longevity greater than that associated with "ideal" or less-than-
"ideal" body weight among persons of middle age and especially among the elderly. The updated 1983 Metropolitan Life
Insurance recommended weights (Metropolitan Life Insurance
Company, 1983) clearly reflect Andres' suggestion. Furthermore, reduction in energy intake automatically reduces the
intake of other macro- and micronutrients, unless very sophisti-
cated and costly changes are made in dietary patterns, resulting
in increases in the nutrient densities of the foods consumed.
Acquiring the sophistication and the funds needed for such
changes is an unlikely voluntary achievement by persons already elderly or aged; hence, finding acceptable methods of
inducing an increase in energy intake is at the top of the rank
order of priorities.

## Fat

Fat is the food with the highest energy density. In today's youth-
oriented culture, fat-containing foods are blacklisted. For the
elderly and aged, however, there is little evidence (Hazzard,
1984) that fat intake has any deleterious effect on cardiovascular
well-being. Augmenting fat intake is an effective means not only
of increasing the energy content but also of increasing the
palatability of diets. Since far more elderly and aged persons are
cachectic than are overweight, the measures commonly used to
induce weight gain among cachectic persons of all ages need to
be applied. One measure frequently recommended to his students by Joseph Aub, a professor at the Harvard Medical School,
is the prescription of butter balls liberally laced with granulated
sugar, a high-energy mixture with exceptional palatability.

## Carbohydrate

Carbohydrate frequently has been condemned as the cause of
everything from drug addiction (Personal papers, 1963) to myocardial infarction, obesity, peptic ulcers, and diabetes (Yudkin,
1963). Carbohydrate intolerance (Andres, 1971, 1981) has been

well documented as an accompaniment of aging that is distinct from that associated with diabetes mellitus. Nonetheless, carbohydrate deserves to be regarded as being more like Cinderella than one of the ugly stepsisters (Passmore, 1964). Carbohydrate is a convenient, relatively inexpensive source of energy. It is a vehicle, depending on its source, of a variety of micronutrients. In some forms (e.g., sucrose and fructose), it imparts great palatability. It has another great virtue: its fiber content. The elderly and the aged need measured quantities of fiber for all the reasons fiber is needed by all others but also for one special reason. The elderly and aged have a high prevalence of diverticulosis. A diet high in fiber results in a bulky fecal mass that requires less pressure to propel than does the fecal mass associated with low-residue diets. The lowered pressure helps protect older persons from ruptures of diverticulae.

## Protein

Although through gluconeogenesis it may be a source of energy, protein should never replace fat and carbohydrate as an energy source for the elderly and the aged. The world literature is replete with disputes (Watkin, 1983) about the protein requirements of older persons. Most studies have been conducted among persons 79 years of age or under, suggesting that relatively little is known about the true needs of persons 80 or over. Hence, the studies among centenarians now being conducted in Kentucky (Thompson et al., 1984) assume particular significance. When intake only is quantified, most studies have suggested that most persons 60 and over are receiving at least two thirds of the Recommended Dietary Allowance (RDA) for protein (Abraham, Carroll, Dresser, & Johnson, 1977a; National Research Council, 1964, 1968, 1974, 1980a; Ohlson et al., 1950; Schlenker, Feurig, Stone, Ohlson, & Mickelson, 1973; Todhunter, 1976). Unfortunately, such studies did not focus on the elderly and the aged. When the dietary intake data for protein accumulated during the Ten-State Nutrition Survey (U.S. Department of Health, Education and Welfare, 1972) are examined, 30.7% of males and 52.8% of females in the low-income states received less than 50 grams of protein from all sources daily. Comparable percentages from the high-income states were 21.4% and 28.9%, respectively. These data suggest that this may be in part an economic issue; however, low-protein diets are found even among those with adequate means. Ideally, elderly and aged persons should consume protein of the highest possible biological value so that the lowest possible excretion of nitrogen by the kidneys would be required. Practically, this is not feasible or mandatory except in managing persons with advanced hepatic or renal disease. A satisfactory compromise is the protein intake proposed in the RDA (National Research Council, 1980a) of 0.8 gm. per kilogram of body weight per day from all sources.

## Calcium

Calcium nutrition concerns the metabolism of bones and teeth, the clotting of blood, and the health of the cardiovascular system. Calcium should be consumed throughout life because of the special role such lifelong intake plays in the prevention and the treatment of osteoporosis. The present decade has seen the development of new interest in the role calcium plays in the physiology and pathology of the cardiovascular system (McCarron et al., 1982), a concern that has been augmented by the introduction of calcium channel blockers in the management of myocardial and vascular disease (American Medical Association, 1983). In spite of this development, calcium's primary role in the battle against aging continues to be its contribution to bone structure. This contribution must begin early in life and must continue throughout life. A major problem today is the low calcium intake in the diets of adolescent women, a result presumably of their fear that dairy products will contribute to weight gain and perhaps due also to the dubious concern that dairy products will contribute to hyperlipidemia. Nonfat dry milk products are widely available and should be consumed by all persons of both sexes, unless there is a very specific, well-confirmed contraindication to milk consumption. In those rare cases, substitute sources of calcium, such as calcium carbonate tablets in quantities not exceeding the RDA for calcium, provide a rational substitute.

The benefits gained by ingestion of adequate quantities of calcium throughout life include protection against fractures from accidents at all ages and particularly against fractures of both cancellous and cortical bone when persons become elderly and aged. However, calcium is not the panacea. For those who have neglected calcium as a dietary component during youth, medical consultation is required. Under appropriate medical management, even those with advanced osteoporosis can be protected from further disability by combinations of calcium, vitamin D, the vitamin D hormone, estrogens and progesterone in women, and well-monitored exercise regimens (Gallagher et al., 1979; Gambrell, 1982; Judd et al., 1981; Riggs et al., 1981; Slovik, Adams, Neer, Holick, & Potts, 1981; Spencer et al., 1984). The reward for such efforts is a reduction in fracture rates and a decrease in the mortality rates from the complications that inevitably accompany the immobilization associated with the treatment of fractures.

## CONCLUSIONS

These brief descriptions of what can be done with fewer than one tenth of the nutrients needed by human beings suggest what can be done to prevent and treat aging when present knowledge of nutrition is combined with modern medical science. But nutrition is more than nutrients enmeshed in scientific medicine. It is the best vehicle currently available for carrying all the resources needed to combat a universal disease. Nutrition is needed by all. It connotes pleasure. It is nonthreatening. It attracts as does a magnet. With over 14,000 NPOA sites now operational, the loci for nutrition, primary health care, education, information and referral, and, if necessary, triage are available. Through them, millions of middle-aged, elderly, and aged Americans are learning how to combat the greatest of the killer diseases—aging itself. NPOA and other organizations like it are a beginning. Their efforts must be assisted by some new attitudes toward aging by young and old. These should include abandonment of the early retirement philosophy, greater emphasis on retraining for new careers and for the continuation of prior careers, and a realization by persons of all ages that, while aging is inevitable, disability and death can be postponed and the years gained be productive and enjoyable if aging is treated in the manner that has enabled this society to overcome the scourges of the past.

Effective longevity is attainable through combining our resources in gerontology, medicine, and nutrition. No one discipline can succeed independently. Nutrition and nutrition programs serve as the most promising vehicles for reaching the desired goal of rectangularizing survival.

# 5
# Nutrition and Bone Loss in Aging

*Herta Spencer*
*Lois Kramer*
*Dace Osis*

The high incidence of osteoporosis in elderly women is a major public health problem because of serious complications that lead to morbidity and require extensive and costly medical care. Osteoporosis is the most common systemic bone disorder in the United States, and this condition affects an estimated 15 to 20 million persons. The incidence of osteoporosis is greater in females than in males, the ratio being 2:1, the incidence being highest in women after the menopause. It is not only hormonal deficiency and aging that lead to bone loss; other factors, including diet, can play an important role in causing bone loss and in intensifying the loss of bone that is expected to occur with aging. Among these factors, the calcium intake over the years appears to play a major role from the preventive point of view.

In many cases, this bone condition is discovered accidentally, during x-ray examination for an unrelated disorder, or it may be detected only after complications occur, for instance a skeletal fracture. In other instances, the physician may suspect or make the diagnosis of osteoporosis but will assume that there is no effective treatment for this disorder. Thus, the patient will be advised that "Nothing can be done, and you'll have to learn to live with it." The diagnosis of osteoporosis and, therefore, its treatment are frequently delayed until this condition is advanced. This is due to the fact that the progression of this bone condition is very gradual and remains asymptomatic for many years (Spencer, 1982).

When the diagnosis of bone loss is finally established roentgenographically osteoporosis will be advanced, because 30% of the bone mineral must be lost before this diagnosis can be made on skeletal x-ray. The vertebral bodies show poor mineralization, they become biconcave, and adjacent vertebrae have a "fish-mouth" appearance. There may be wedging of the vertebrae resulting in vertebral compression. Thoraco-lumbar vertebrae are frequently involved. These changes in the bone structure in osteoporosis are usually associated with loss of body height, kyphosis, deformity of the chest, and the presence of a "dowager's hump."

Routine x-rays of the skeleton are not reliable indicators of bone density because of differences in techniques and subjective interpretations of x-ray findings. Newer, more reliable methods are available for making the diagnosis of osteoporosis more precisely and earlier than conventional radiographs. These newer methods for determining bone density are photon absorptiometry and the cortical index. Photon absorptiometry (Mazess, 1982) is not routinely done because the equipment is available only in certain centers. Cortical index measurements can be determined by analyzing an x-ray of the hand, which is done by relating the cortical thickness to the total width of the metacarpal bone. Another method for determining bone density is radiographic absorptiometry, which utilizes radiographs of the hands and a computer scanner (Colbert & Bachtell, 1981). Bone biopsies (needle biopsies) are desirable for establishing the diagnosis of osteoporosis objectively, but this technique is invasive and is not acceptable to many patients.

Factors that can contribute to the development of calcium loss are certain dietary factors as well as the use of several drugs. With regard to the dietary factors, a low calcium intake consumed over prolonged periods of time (years) has an adverse effect on calcium metabolism. The interaction of calcium with other minerals also has to be considered in terms of absorption and utilization of calcium. In addition, drugs as well as the long-term excessive use of alcohol can induce significant calcium loss resulting in bone loss and in changes of the bone structure. The combined use of drugs and the long-term excess use of alcohol are expected to have an intensifying effect on increasing the calcium loss. It is well known that exercise is an important factor in maintaining the normal bone structure and that severe bone loss, even in young persons, can be induced by immobilization, the bone loss in paraplegia being an extreme example of this effect.

We now will discuss some of the dietary factors that have to be considered in maintaining the skeletal structure.

## CALCIUM INTAKE

The recommended dietary intake of calcium in the United States is 800 mg/day (National Research Council, 1980a). It is, however, highly relevant to examine whether this amount of calcium is adequate throughout adult life for maintaining the normal skeletal structure and for preventing bone loss in later life with aging, particularly in females. The intake of adequate calcium throughout adult life appears to play an important role, as it has been shown that a person's peak bone mass is achieved by age 30 to 35 and declines thereafter. This decrease in bone mass is then accelerated in females after the menopause. One may therefore safely assume that the inevitable bone loss due to increased bone resorption in later life can be minimized by building a strong skeleton at an early age. Also, there are statements in the literature that persons who have been diagnosed to have osteoporosis have had a low dietary calcium intake over the years. In view of the calcium loss with aging, particularly in women, it has been recommended that the calcium intake of postmenopausal women should be considerably greater than 800 mg/day and that it should in fact be increased to 1500 mg/day (Heaney, Recker, & Saville, 1977). An increase in calcium intake over and above the 800 mg/day can be achieved by increasing the intake of dairy products. If for any reason dairy products are not well tolerated, calcium supplements may be added, such as calcium carbonate, calcium gluconate, or calcium lactate.

There is a general belief that adaptation to a low-calcium

intake occurs (Draper & Scythes, 1981); however, other investigators have reported just the reverse (Allen, 1982; Heaney et al., 1982). We have observed in our extensive long-term studies that there is no adaptation to a low-calcium intake with time, irrespective of the duration of an inadequate, very low dietary intake of calcium (Spencer & Kramer, 1985). The calcium balance remained as negative after several months of this low calcium intake as in the initial phase. We also have observed that the intestinal absorption of calcium does not increase with time during a prolonged low-calcium intake, in order to compensate for the long-term insufficient supply of calcium. This has been conclusively demonstrated in $Ca^{47}$ absorption studies that were carried out with subjects having a constant calcium intake (Spencer & Kramer, 1985).

With regard to the recommended dietary calcium intake of 800 mg/day, extensive studies have shown that the calcium balances were negative during this calcium intake in a large percentage of the persons studied, indicating that variable amounts of calcium continue to be lost daily at a calcium intake of 800 mg/day (Spencer et al., 1984). At a higher calcium intake of 1200 mg/day, the calcium balance becomes more positive and a plateau of the calcium balance was reached. Furthermore, increasing the calcium intake beyond this level, up to 2200 mg/day, had no effect on increasing the retention of calcium more than during a calcium intake of 1200 mg/day. In view of the plateau of the calcium balance reached at the 1200-mg/day level, and the negative calcium balances observed during the 800-mg/day level, it appears that the recommended intake of calcium should be greater than 800 mg/day. This aspect is stressed because practically 100% of persons who had osteoporosis showed negative calcium balances at the 800-mg/day level. In view of the fact that bone loss in osteoporosis is a very gradual process that may extend over many years before it is clinically demonstrable, it would be preferable to recommend a higher calcium intake than 800 mg/day, although there is no definite proof for the calcium-deficiency etiology of osteoporosis.

Table 5.1 shows the calcium balances determined in 108 studies involving different intake levels of calcium. With a low calcium intake of approximately 200 mg/day, the calcium bal-

## TABLE 5.1
### Calcium and Phosphorus Balances at Different Calcium Intakes

| Study | No. of Studies | Average Study/Days | Calcium (mg/day) | | | | Phosphorus (mg/day) | | | | Ca/P Ratio |
|---|---|---|---|---|---|---|---|---|---|---|---|
| | | | Intake | Urine | Stool | Balance | Intake | Urine | Stool | Balance | |
| **Calcium intake, 200 mg/day** | | | | | | | | | | | |
| Low Calcium | 22 | 37 | 234 | 85 | 244 | −95 | 833 | 554 | 255 | +74 | 1/4 |
| SEM | | | ±6 | ±10 | ±16 | ±15 | ±23 | ±30 | ±9 | ±20 | |
| **Calcium intake, 800 mg/day** | | | | | | | | | | | |
| Calcium gluconate | 67 | 36 | 804 | 178 | 603 | +22 | 857 | 525 | 298 | +34 | 1/1 |
| SEM | | | ±6 | ±11 | ±13 | ±8 | ±16 | ±14 | ±7 | ±9 | |
| **Calcium intake, 1200 mg/day** | | | | | | | | | | | |
| Calcium gluconate | 7 | 29 | 1230 | 166 | 958 | +106 | 861 | 464 | 295 | +101 | 1.5/1 |
| SEM | | | ±13 | ±46 | ±39 | ±46 | ±49 | ±45 | ±13 | ±27 | |
| **Calcium intake, 2000 mg/day** | | | | | | | | | | | |
| Calcium gluconate | 12 | 34 | 2021 | 150 | 1724 | +147 | 801 | 338 | 328 | +135 | 2.5/1 |
| SEM | | | ±14 | ±20 | ±41 | ±32 | ±15 | ±26 | ±11 | ±26 | |

ance was negative, as expected. Increasing the calcium intake fourfold to about 800 mg/day resulted in a slightly positive calcium balance, +22 mg/day. Increasing the calcium intake further to about 1200 mg/day resulted in a more positive calcium balance, +106 mg/day. The level of the calcium balance did not significantly increase further when the calcium intake was increased by an additional 800 mg to a total of 2000 mg/day.

## PHOSPHORUS INTAKE

The American diet is generally alleged to have a very high phosphorus content, which has been alleged to have adverse effects on calcium metabolism and on bone. However, the usual dietary phosphorus intake is approximately 1200 mg/day. Strictly controlled studies have shown that increasing the phosphorus intake further, up to 2000 mg/day, had no adverse effect on the calcium status. This was true both when a high phosphorus intake of 2000 mg per day was combined with a low calcium intake of 200 mg/day as well as when it was paired with a high calcium intake of 2000 mg/day (see Table 5.2). In fact, the high phosphorus intake has a desirable effect in that it leads to a decrease of the urinary calcium (Spencer, Menczel, Lewin, & Samachson, 1965; Spencer, Kramer, Osis, & Norris, 1978a; Goldsmith & Ingbar, 1966). Our studies have shown that this beneficial effect of added phosphorus can be observed at any level of calcium intake; that is, a definite decrease of the urinary calcium can be achieved. In line with these observations are reports that have shown that phosphorus supplements also have the beneficial effect of aiding in fracture healing (Goldsmith & Ingbar, 1966).

## PROTEIN INTAKE

The usual dietary intake of protein is approximately 1 gm protein per kg body weight per day. There is a widespread belief

TABLE 5.2
Effect of Phosphorus on the Calcium Balance
During Different Calcium Intakes

| No. of Studies | Study Days | Phosphorus Intake,[a] mg/day | Calcium mg/day[a] | | | |
|---|---|---|---|---|---|---|
| | | | Intake | Urine | Stool | Balance |
| 7 | 36 | 797 | 230 | 137 | 193 | −100 |
| | | ±30[b] | ±13 | ±22 | ±27 | ±35 |
| | 32 | 1993 | 230 | 57 | 265 | −92 |
| | | ±5 | ±11 | ±14 | ±26 | ±24 |
| 8 | 40 | 765 | 2028 | 216 | 1569 | +243 |
| | | ±26 | ±29 | ±38 | ±60 | ±30 |
| | 36 | 1965 | 1993 | 135 | 1609 | +252 |
| | | ±22 | ±17 | ±26 | ±46 | ±22 |

[a]All values are averages for the number of studies and for the number of study days.
[b]SEM = Standard error of the Mean.

that a high protein intake has deleterious effects on calcium metabolism, in that it increases urinary calcium and induces calcium loss. It should be emphasized, however, that this calciuric effect of a high protein intake is usually observed when using purified proteins such as casein, lactalbumin, gelatin, egg-white, and a wide variety of amino acids (Linkswiler, Joyce, & Anand, 1974; Margen, Chu, Kaufmann, & Calloway, 1974). These isolated protein fractions are usually not consumed alone but are contained in the human diet in a complex form with other nutrients. The main sources of dietary protein are meat and dairy products. In our research studies, a high protein intake, given as meat, did not increase the urinary excretion of calcium in a large number of cases (Spencer, Kramer, DeBartolo, Norris, & Osis, 1983; Spencer, Kramer, Osis, & Norris, 1978b). Table 5.3 shows calcium balance data determined in three studies carried out during high protein intake of 2 gm protein per kg body weight per day. This high protein intake, given as meat, did not result in any significant increase in urinary calcium or fecal

## TABLE 5.3
### Effect of a High Protein (Meat) Intake on the Calcium Balance and on the Intestinal Absorption of Calcium

| Patient | Study | Study Days | Protein (g/kg) | Calcium (mg/day) | | | | $Ca^{47}$ Absorption % |
|---|---|---|---|---|---|---|---|---|
| | | | | Intake | Urine | Stool | Balance | |
| 1 | Control | 30 | 1.0 | 217 | 93 | 218 | −94 | 59 |
| | High Protein[a] | 36 | 2.0 | 205 | 110[b] | 177 | −82 | 61 |
| 2 | Control | 24 | 1.0 | 805 | 119 | 743 | −57 | 54 |
| | High Protein[a] | 90 | 2.0 | 833 | 105 | 739 | −11 | 55 |
| 3 | Control | 24 | 1.0 | 1113 | 69 | 863 | +181 | 30 |
| | High Protein[a] | 42 | 2.0 | 1109 | 50 | 849 | +210 | 25 |

[a]High protein intake given as red meat.
[b]Not significant.

calcium, and the calcium balance did not change, even when the high protein intake was given for as long as 90 days. Also, there was no change of the intestinal absorption of calcium.

## EFFECT OF DRUGS ON CALCIUM METABOLISM

It is usually not appreciated that commonly used medications can induce an increase in the excretion of calcium and that, if used for a prolonged period of time, these drugs may induce significant calcium loss. This calcium loss may contribute to or intensify an already existing low calcium status, as is the case in postmenopausal osteoporosis. Among these drugs, corticosteroids and thyroid medications are the ones commonly known to cause calcium loss and to lead to the development of osteoporosis; however, other medications can have a similar effect. Examples of these are the long-term use of the antibiotic tetracycline and the long-term use of the antituberculous drug isoniazid (INH) (Spencer, Kramer, & Osis, 1982). Also, certain diuretics, such as the commonly used drug furosemide (Lasix), have been shown to induce an increase of the urinary calcium excretion.

Among the commonly used drugs that induce considerable calcium loss are the aluminum-containing antacids. The use of these drugs has an adverse effect on bone and when used for prolonged periods of time can lead to the development of osteoporosis. The primary effect of these antacids is the inhibition of the intestinal absorption of phosphorus by aluminum, resulting in phosphorus depletion. The phosphorus depletion by aluminum, which is caused by complexation of phosphorus by aluminum in the intestine, results in a secondary loss of calcium which is reflected by the increased excretion of calcium in both urine and stool. This increase in calcium excretion results in a negative calcium balance. Even relatively small doses of these antacids can induce these adverse effects (Spencer, Kramer, Norris, & Osis, 1982), and the calcium loss is further intensified by the use of large therapeutic doses (Lotz, Zisman, & Bartter, 1968; Spencer, Kramer, Norris, & Osis, 1982). Figure 5.1 shows an example of the negative calcium balance induced by small doses of aluminum hydroxide.

Table 5.4 shows data obtained in studies carried out in two patients by Spencer, Kramer, Norris, and Osis (1982) on the effect of large doses of aluminum-containing antacids. The dose of the antacid was 450 ml/day. The main effect was the high excretion of phosphorus in stool and the extremely low urinary excretion of phosphorus. The adverse effects of the aluminum-containing antacids on calcium metabolism are reflected by the increase of both the urinary and fecal calcium excretion, resulting in a markedly negative calcium balance, the calcium loss being 250 and 502 mg/day, for the two patients, respectively. Extensive calcium loss, evidenced on bone x-rays, has been seen in fully ambulatory male patients who have used aluminum-containing antacids for several years.

Although alcohol is not classified as a drug, it should be emphasized that the long-term use of excessive alcohol has an adverse effect on bone. The reason for the bone loss in chronic alcoholism is difficult to identify, as many factors may play a

**FIGURE 5.1   Effect of Aluminum Hydroxide on Phosphorus and Calcium Balances**

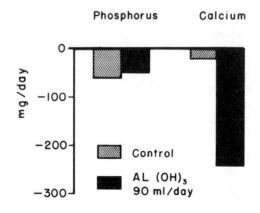

## TABLE 5.4
### Effect of Large Doses of Maalox on Mineral Metabolism

| Patient | Study | Antacid ml/day | Study Days | Calcium (mg/day) | | | | Phosphorus (mg/day) | | | |
|---|---|---|---|---|---|---|---|---|---|---|---|
| | | | | Intake | Urine | Stool | Balance | Intake | Urine | Stool | Balance |
| 1 | Maalox | 450 | 12 | 346 | 209 | 394 | −257 | 1007 | 13 | 1148 | −154 |
| | Post–Maalox | | 18 | 219 | 76 | 165 | −22 | 908 | 510 | 207 | +191 |
| 2 | Control | | 18 | 253 | 82 | 348 | −177 | 922 | 482 | 285 | +156 |
| | Maalox | 450 | 12 | 279 | 421 | 360 | −502 | 873 | 18 | 890 | −35 |

83

role, such as insufficient intake of dietary calcium, protein, and vitamin D. Other factors may be steatorrhea, as well as the intake of aluminum-containing antacids to alleviate symptoms of alcoholic gastritis. Extensive bone loss and osteoporosis, proven on bone biopsy, have been observed in relatively young and middle-aged fully ambulatory males with chronic alcoholism. No other cause other than chronic alcoholism could be identified for the calcium loss in these patients (Spencer, Rubio, Rubio, Indreika, & Seitam, in press).

# 6

# Nutrition and the Elderly: Selected Social, Cultural, and Economic Issues

*Cary S. Kart*

National studies dating back almost 20 years to the Department of Agriculture's Household Food Consumption Survey in 1965 indicate a substantial proportion of the U.S. aged population to be nutritionally vulnerable. A large number of the aged consume diets that are insufficient in calories and deficient in nutrients necessary for maintaining physical health and well-being. Those particularly vulnerable would seem to be the low-income aged and those who are sick and disabled. The national surveys (including the Ten-State Nutrition Survey and HANES) also have shown that many of the aged are consuming diets wholly inappropriate as therapeutic regimens for managing acute or chronic diseases (Barrows & Roeder, 1977; Kart & Metress, 1984).

Data from a wide array of regional and local nutrition studies corroborate findings from the national surveys in that they broadly define the scope of nutritional vulnerability among the elderly. In addition, these local studies further emphasize the complexity of factors that may interact to affect the food intake and nutritional status of the aged. These include socioeconomic considerations such as income and education, sex, living arrangements, and the availability of meal programs to supplement dietary intake. O'Hanlon and Kohrs (1978) provide a summary of approximately 25 local and regional dietary studies of older Americans.

Traditionally, the factors that affect the nutritional status of the elderly have been divided into two broad groups: (1) those that result from metabolic and physiological changes associated with aging; and (2) those that affect the amount and type of food eaten. This latter group includes social, cultural, and economic factors, which are probably the most important influences on eating habits at any age. The emphasis in this chapter is on this latter group, though I would like to make a further division or refinement in this category. This refinement reflects the distinction a methodologist might make among or between units of analysis. In the first part of this chapter, I want to emphasize the individual as the unit of analysis and briefly (and in general terms) describe some adjustments many older people are forced to make which have impact on nutritional status. In particular, these adjustments reflect the economic deprivation suffered by many of the aged. In the latter part, I want to consider the society as the unit of analysis and suggest that both the current public policy and the medical-legal environments may have decidedly negative implications for the nutritional status of older people. In particular, I look first to the continuing and perhaps increasing unlikelihood of any national nutrition policy initiatives to fight hunger and malnutrition among the elderly (or anyone else, for that matter). Then I will examine a recent state appellate court decision that may have profound impact on the nutritional status of older people, especially the most vulnerable elderly.

## NUTRITIONAL ADJUSTMENTS OF OLDER PEOPLE

Those who work with the elderly often come to realize that metabolic and physiological barriers to proper nutrition may be minor compared to those factors that actually regulate food intake (Kart & Metress, 1984). Factors governing food intake determine the quantity, quality, and combinations of food eaten; they are intricately interwoven into the fabric of the elderly person's social life. As is the case for people of all ages, food can be as important to the elderly for social and psychological reasons as it is for physiological well-being. I wish to make only fleeting reference here to the symbolic content of eating and feeding in this society and the association of food with caring and comfort, a theme I will return to later in this chapter.

The sociocultural factors that affect food intake are quite varied. Each elderly person is the product of years of experience in a social and cultural setting modified by individual perception and choice. As a result, long-standing dietary habits and ideas can be difficult to change. Dietary habits are often carried from youth, associated with what Capron (1984) describes as primal parent–child relations. As a result, they may take on increased significance with age. Because of such enduring habits and attached sentiment, people often seem to prefer or reject certain foods in the face of direct evidence that such foods are good or bad for them.

Income is a primary factor in determining diet at all ages. Many gerontologists believe that the major problems of geriatric nutrition are a function not of age but rather of the socioeconomic status of the aged (Watkin, 1983). My summary of the findings of recent national nutrition surveys would suggest they are right (Kart & Metress, 1984). Retirement income, in comparison with preretirement earnings, is reduced for the great majority of older people. Although several experts have agreed that 65 to 80% of preretirement earnings is required by retirees (Munnell, 1977; Schulz et al., 1974), a recent study reports that median Social Security replacement rates for retirees during the mid-1970s varied between 32 and 49% (Munnell, 1977). For many of those described by Nelson (1982) as "downwardly mobile" elderly, Social Security represents the principal, if not only, source of retirement income.

As a result, poverty is a fact of life for many elderly, especially nonwhite aged. As Table 6.1 shows, approximately 15% of the 1982 aged population is impoverished and almost 4 out of 10

**TABLE 6.1**
**Poverty Rates: 1959, 1968, 1977, & 1982**

|                        | Percent Living in Poverty | | | |
|------------------------|------|------|------|------|
|                        | 1959 | 1968 | 1977 | 1982 |
| Total population       | 22   | 13   | 12   | 15   |
| Total aged population  | 35   | 25   | 14   | 15   |
| Whites                 | 33   | 23   | 12   | 12   |
| Nonwhites              | 61   | 47   | 35   | 38   |

*Source:* Based on data from the U.S. Bureau of the Census, *Current Population Reports,* Series P-60, No. 116 (1978) and No. 140 (1983).

nonwhite elderly have incomes below the poverty level. This is particularly telling as the so-called "poverty index" is based on the amount of money needed to purchase a minimum adequate diet as determined by the Department of Agriculture. Actually, using consumer expenditure surveys completed in the late 1950s that showed food to account for approximately one third of a household budget, the poverty index is calculated at *three times* the cost of the minimum adequate food diet. For example, in 1982 the poverty-level income for a single person aged 65 or over was approximately $4,600, while that for an aged couple was about $5,800 (derivative poverty income cutoff points are estimated for families of differing size and composition with a farm/nonfarm differential for each family type).

Critics believe that the poverty index severely underestimates poverty. Consumer expenditure surveys completed in the 1960s and 1970s show food to constitute about 20 percent of a household budget (see Table 6.2). Thus, a poverty index calculated at *five times* the cost of the minimum adequate food diet would seem in order (U.S. Department of Health, Education and Welfare, 1976). This formula would have raised the 1982 poverty-level income for a single aged person to about $7,700 and for an aged couple to about $9,700, a 67-percent increase in each case. Further, the current poverty index uses a measure of adequate diet based on the Department of Agriculture's 1963 Economy Food Plan. In 1975 this food plan was replaced with a new Thrifty Food Plan reflecting revised allowances for essential nutrients and newer data on family food choices. Experts suggest that basing the poverty index on the new food plan (without altering the formula for computing the poverty level from a 3:1 to a 5:1 ratio) would increase the poverty threshold by about 40 percent above the current levels (Orshansky, 1978). By itself, this should approximately double the number of aged poor to include almost one in three Americans 65 years of age or older. As an aside, the poverty index is not applied to the "hidden poor," those who are institutionalized or living with relatives (Orshansky, 1978).

Housing, health care, transportation, and other expenses compete with food expenses. Table 6.2 compares the operating expenses of households having a family head under age 65 with those in which the family head is 65 years or over. When compared with younger families, families headed by an aged

**TABLE 6.2**
**Operating Expenses: A Comparison by Age Group**

| Expense | Percent of Household Income | |
|---|---|---|
| | Family Head under 65 | Family Head 65 and Over |
| Housing | 26.0 | 28.9 |
| Food | 18.2 | 21.4 |
| Health care | 4.8 | 8.3 |
| Clothing | 7.3 | 5.4 |
| Furniture and household equipment | 4.4 | 3.2 |
| Recreation | 7.1 | 6.2 |
| Alcohol and tobacco | 2.3 | 1.7 |
| Transportation | 17.9 | 12.8 |
| Other (gifts, contributions, personal care, etc.) | 12.0 | 12.1 |

*Source*: H. B. Brotman (1978). The aging of America: A demographic profile. *National Journal, 10*(40), 1622–1627. Reprinted by permission.

person are found to spend a greater proportion of their income on housing, food, and health care.

Because of insufficient purchasing power, many elderly shoppers cannot buy food on the basis of past eating habits or recommended daily allowances of nutrients. They develop a tendency to purchase cheaper foods high in refined carbohydrates, such as bread and cereals, rather than more expensive protective foods such as meat, fruit, and vegetables. It is not the carbohydrates per se that are bad, but the lack of dietary variety fostered by such purchasing patterns. Reduced variety often leads to reduced quality and increased risk of malnutrition.

The elderly, like the poor in general, are often forced to shop at more expensive stores in the absence of chain stores in the neighborhood or because of a lack of transportation to volume-sale stores with lower prices. Alternatively, the need to obtain credit to purchase food between retirement checks may arise. This may necessitate the use of "Ma and Pa" grocery stores that give credit but must charge higher prices and carry a smaller variety of products than chain stores.

The aged are often unable to take advantage of sales or quantity discounts because they lack proper storage facilities including refrigeration and pest-free cupboards. Many a middle-class geriatric nutritionist has taken for granted conveniences not always available to the poor and/or elderly. If money is not available for food at the time of the month when sales occur, the bargains are unobtainable. Food activist groups have observed deliberate price inflation of food products at the time of the month when welfare and Social Security checks arrive. The poor do pay more, and, as we have already seen, a significant proportion of the elderly are poor.

Modern marketing procedures are geared toward the younger consumer with a family. The elderly, especially those who live alone or have storage problems, need smaller quantities of food. Yet small quantities are often unavailable or, if available, are more expensive than the same foods bought in larger amounts. The trend toward prepackaging perishables creates problems for the elderly. The quantities prepackaged are often aimed at families, not single marketers. Furthermore, food packaging itself presents a challenge. Elderly individuals with failing vision, waning strength, and/or declining fine coordination may be frustrated by such packaging materials. Marketing techniques aimed at higher profits, including end-of-aisle displays and multiple-item pricing, affect both young and old. But many elderly have less margin for error in budgeting their limited funds.

Eating is part of the complex arrangements of interpersonal interaction and, as such, has significant social and psychological impact on the elderly individual. Food can be a great comfort during times of loss, such as the death of spouse or companion, or even in the face of loss of social involvements. Losses force rearrangement of the individual's social world and upset balances. Reestablishment of the old balance or creation of a new one may be difficult. Foods associated with significant events and periods in the lives of old people and their loved ones may be helpful in readjusting the individual's world.

Loss of a spouse can be a special source of dietary stress. The majority of aged women are widows; they outnumber widowers by a ratio of about 5:1. Although widowers remarry at a substantially higher rate than widows, those who do not may have special difficulty in adjusting. The few studies of widowers indicate that their main problems include loneliness and discomfort over self-maintenance tasks, for example, Berardo (1970). Widowers are often unable to take care of their own basic needs, especially if they have been married since youth and were dependent upon their wives for socialization. Because of this, some of the worst nutritional problems often occur among elderly widowers. Widows, on the other hand, seem able to continue to perform domestic tasks that an elderly male never learned to do, but they are more likely to find themselves in financial distress (Atchley, 1975). In addition, if her spouse had functioned as the money manager throughout the marriage, a new widow may be unable to cope with even simple household management problems.

In the United States, the role of older widow is an ambiguous one. In fact, there are no clear expectations for behavior in this role. Given the anomic situation in which older widows find themselves, it is no wonder that the great bulk of research on widowhood highlights the negative personal consequences that accompany the change from spouse to widow. Statistics indicate that the widowed have higher rates of mortality, mental disorders, and suicide (Berardo, 1968; Riley & Foner, 1968). It has generally been assumed that widowhood brings low morale (Atchley, 1975). Shulman (1975) has reported that widows are more likely than single or married elderly to describe the past as the happiest time of life and are twice as likely to be depressed or lonely.

Loss of companionship can seriously affect an individual's motivation to shop, cook, eat, remain active, or even go on living. It also may reduce physical activity and/or social participation that previously diverted attention from personal problems.

Emotional stress can cause a loss of appetite and the development of negative protein, calcium, and magnesium balances because of increased excretion associated with stress (Altschule, 1978; Scrimshaw, 1964). Stress also can lead to compulsive eating and the onset of obesity, which may further complicate health problems associated with old age. The elderly person who feels rejected or neglected by his or her own family and friends may use eating as an attention-getting device.

Finally, a number of basic logistical problems affect the ability of the elderly to get enough to eat. Lack of adequate cooking facilities may be a problem for those living in low-cost rentals and single-room-occupancy hotels. Old and sometimes dangerous cooking or kitchen utensils may discourage use. One solution in such circumstances is avoidance of meal preparation.

## NATIONAL NUTRITION POLICY: A DIM VISION

The popular political ideology that views federal involvement in social and health programs in negative terms may be strong evidence that the likelihood of achieving a broad agreement on a national nutrition policy is at best a dim vision of some possible future (Kart & Metress, 1984). Still, this reactionary political ideology does not deserve all the blame. The concern and debate over national nutrition policy has been with us for at least a generation. It is now 20 years since the pilot Food Stamp Program, initiated by executive order of President Kennedy in 1961, was institutionalized in the Food Stamp Act of 1964. This legislation represented a compromise between proponents of a food program for the poor and the interests of agricultural producers (Schmandt, Shorey, & Kinch, 1980). In the period since, a variety of additional and highly successful food programs has been created, including senior nutrition programs and home-delivered meals in the Older Americans Act, School Breakfast, Child Food, Summer Food, WIC (Special Supplemental Food Program for Women, Infants and Children), and NET (Nutrition Education and Training Program). This latter group, of course, is aimed primarily at the young.

This collection of programs hardly represents a concerted systematic federal attack on hunger and malnutrition in the United States. Ten years ago, the National Nutrition Consortium developed five general goals to be included in a national nutrition policy (U.S. Senate, 1974a). These are as follows:

1. Assure an adequate wholesome food supply at reasonable cost to meet the needs of all segments of the population. This supply is to be available at a level consistent with the affordable lifestyle of the era.
2. Maintain food resources sufficient to meet emergency needs, and fulfill a responsible role as a nation in meeting world food needs.
3. Develop a level of sound public knowledge and responsible understanding of nutrition and foods that will promote maximal nutritional knowledge.
4. Maintain a system of quality and safety control that justifies public confidence in its food supply.
5. Support research and education in foods and nutrition with adequate resources and reasoned priorities to solve important content problems and to permit exploratory basic research.

These goals, abstract as they are, seem as pertinent today as they were 10 years ago. Yet, even in the presence of a more accepting political ideology than now exists, implementation would be difficult. Balkanization of responsibilities and authorities is one serious barrier to this effort. Currently, there is no single office that administers the federal machinery for food and nutrition. Four additional reasons for the lack of action on a national nutrition policy seem apparent.

## Low Federal Priority

First, it would seem that nutrition is a low federal priority. This may be especially the case today in an administration whose highest officials believe that soup kitchens are being used by the well-to-do to avoid paying for meals. Remember, President Reagan's Task Force on Food Assistance asserted that it was impossible to estimate the extent of hunger in America, anyway, and, further, that "people in need of food assistance would benefit if the programs or any subset of them were controlled at a more local level, such as the state or county" (Parker, 1984, pp. 7–11). This would imply that basic nutritional needs vary from locality to locality!

Still, the low federal priority assigned to nutrition programs has been with us for a while. In 1973, President Nixon directed every major department and agency to define its high-priority objectives. Early in 1974, 144 federal objectives received presidential approval. Two of these were concerned with nutrition: (1) the "development of a cost-effective child nutrition program" and (2) the "rationalization [justifying] of eligibility requirements for food stamps." Notice the absence of mentioned objectives aimed specifically at the elderly.

## Nutrition as Welfare Policy Rather Than Health Policy

The second reason for lack of action is that the preeminent policy viewpoint in the federal government seems to associate nutrition with "income maintenance" programs rather than with health policies. For example, the 1975 presidential budget message proposed the "transfer of food stamps and related nutrition programs to the Department of HEW to improve coordination of income maintenance programs." This emphasis on income maintenance continues. The President's Task Force on Food Assistance, mentioned earlier, has recommended including the value of "in-kind" benefits like food stamps as income, as a solution to the relationship between poverty, hunger, and malnutrition. The President's Private Sector Survey on Cost Control (PPSS)—sometimes referred to as the Grace Commission Report, after its chairman J. Peter Grace—has also recommended including in-kind benefits such as food stamps in cash-in-means testing to determine eligibility for any number of other federal program benefits. The White House Office of Management and Budget estimates that, by adding the cash value of noncash benefits (e.g., food stamps, health care benefits, housing subsidies, and the like) to other sources of income, the reported poverty rate in 1982 would have dropped from 15 to 9.6%.

This accounting change would reduce the poverty rate by more than one third and commensurately deny to a significant proportion of the most needy any access to governmental programs. Many of the elderly poor receive noncash benefits from a variety of sources. Counting health benefits as income, for example, may act to deny eligibility for food stamps and housing subsidies. Interestingly, the Grace Commission Report does point to the substantial savings already accruing to the federal government from the large numbers of elderly who are eligible for participation in the Food Stamp Program but who do not participate. One recent study of households comprised entirely of persons 65 years or older and screened for Food Stamp Program eligibility estimated overall participation rates to range from 43 to 59% (Hollonbeck & Ohls, 1984). Substantial numbers of households in this study cited the belief that they were ineligible as a reason for nonparticipation; many indicated they "didn't need" the benefits or that the benefits "didn't seem worth the trouble." Stigma or embarrassment about receiving the benefits was also an important deterrent to participation (Hollonbeck & Ohls, 1984). Grace and his colleagues did not make recommendations to the federal government on how best to increase the participation rates in the Food Stamp Program of the eligible elderly.

## Lack of Governmental Understanding

Third, the poor quality of the government's information on the status of nutrition and health probably precludes any breakthrough in national nutrition policy. It is fragmentary, partial, and sometimes improvised (U.S. Senate, 1974b). In part, this results from the Balkanization of responsibilities; no single focus exists in the executive branch of government for assessing and advocating nutrition policies.

## Difficulty of Achieving Broad Agreement

Finally, the lack of action on national nutrition policy also has to do with the difficulty of achieving broad agreement among nutrition experts about public policy issues. A consideration of the proposed dietary goals for the United States should exemplify this problem. In 1977, the U.S. Senate Select Committee on Nutrition and Human Needs proposed a set of dietary goals for the United States. These goals, listed in Table 6.3, were not viewed as a panacea for disease, but rather as healthful guides to follow. In part they represented an outgrowth of concern that dietary changes occurring in the United States since the beginning of this century pose a significant threat to the nation's health. The Senate Committee, while recognizing the existence of malnutrition, argued that the major dietary concern for the United States as a whole is the problem of "overnutrition"— eating too much of the wrong foods. It noted that 6 of the 10 leading causes of death in the United States, including heart disease, cancer, and stroke, have been linked to diet.

The Senate's dietary goals were firmly endorsed by prominent nutrition and health authorities. Despite the endorsements, there was considerable controversy over the goals, even within the nutrition establishment. One concern involved the state of scientific evidence on the relationship between nutrition and disease. Some believed the evidence to be insufficiently complete to warrant making recommendations to the public. An emphasis on the goals without any significant improvement in the incidence of disease might undermine confidence in profes-

**TABLE 6.3**
**U.S. Dietary Goals, 1977**

1. To avoid overweight, consume only as much energy as is expended; if overweight, decrease energy intake and increase energy expenditure.
2. Increase the consumption of complex carbohydrates and "naturally occurring" sugars from about 28 percent of energy intake to about 48 percent of energy intake.
3. Reduce the consumption of refined and processed sugars by about 45 percent to account for about 10 percent of total energy intake.
4. Reduce overall fat consumption from approximately 40 percent to about 30 percent of energy intake.
5. Reduce saturated fat consumption to account for about 10 percent of total energy intake, and balance that with polyunsaturated and monosaturated fats, which should account for about 10 percent of energy intake each.
6. Reduce cholesterol consumption to about 300 mg/day.
7. Limit the intake of sodium by reducing the intake of salt to about 5 gm/day.

*Source*: U.S. Senate Select Committee on Nutrition and Human Needs. (1977). *Dietary Goals for the United States*, 2nd ed. Washington, DC: U.S. Government Printing Office.

sional advice concerning health habits. More specifically, nutrition science might suffer if future research indicated the need for a *new* set of dietary goals. Later advice might also be ignored if the stated goals appeared unjustifiable.

The concerns of some of these critics were clearly a consequence of economic considerations. As Caliendo (1981) has pointed out, the institutionalization of the goals could have dramatic economic repercussions. If the demand for food shifts from animal and dairy products, for example, to more fresh produce and whole-grain products, there could be severe economic problems for the dairy and meat sectors.

In 1980, the U.S. Department of Agriculture and what is now the U.S. Department of Health and Human Services reacted to the controversy over the goals by publishing a more general set of dietary guidelines:

1. Eat a variety of food daily.
2. Maintain ideal weight.
3. Avoid too much fat, unsaturated fat, and cholesterol.
4. Eat foods with adequate starch and fiber.
5. Avoid too much sugar.
6. Avoid too much sodium.
7. If you drink alcohol, do so in moderation.

But even then the controversy did not die. The Food and Nutrition Board (National Research Council, 1980b) published a report entitled *Toward Healthful Diets.* This report deviated from the dietary guidelines just listed in the areas of fat, cholesterol, and carbohydrates in the diet. For example, the Food and Nutrition Board (FNB) said that only people at risk for heart disease should worry about cholesterol. (This was despite the fact that a recent National Institutes of Health conference cited numerous scientific studies that established what was termed a "cause-and-effect" relationship between high blood cholesterol and heart attacks. Importantly, the conference recommended that the entire U.S. population, except for children under age 2, follow a low-fat, low-cholesterol diet.) The FNB also remarked that only obese individuals and those at risk of heart disease should be concerned about fat and only diabetics should be concerned about fat and the mix of sugars and complex carbohydrates (Hitt, 1982).

Interestingly, both the USDA/USDHHS and the FNB guidelines were based on an examination of similar if not the same scientific evidence. What accounts for the differences in recommendations? One explanation is that, whereas the government looked at the total population and what could be done to improve the health of people in general, the FNB seems to have approached the matter clinically, as a physician would treat a single patient (Hitt, 1982). The incompleteness of scientific evidence on the relationship between nutrition and health and the lack of agreement as to what constitutes appropriate dietary goals or guidelines for the U.S. population would seem to indicate that formulation of a national nutrition policy is a very remote possibility.

# IN THE MATTER OF MARY HIER

Are feeding and hydration medical treatments? The answer to this question could have profound impact on the nutritional status of the most vulnerable elderly. Several recent state appellate and supreme court decisions have dealt with the rights of elderly incompetents to have (or be denied) access to food and water. In this section we discuss the case of Mary Hier (464 N.E. 2d 959, Mass. App. 1984), an aged and ill nursing home patient who was being fed through the surgical implantation of a feeding tube directly into her stomach.

At the time of these proceedings, Mary Hier was a 92-year-old mentally ill woman who had been a resident of a psychiatric hospital in New York State for 57 years. She was transferred to a nursing home in Massachusetts in October of 1983. Both in New York and again in Massachusetts she had received Thorazine to relieve her delusions and extreme agitation. For many years, she also had suffered from a hiatal hernia and a large cervical diverticulum in her esophagus, the combined effect of which was to impede greatly her ability to ingest food. In 1974, in New York, she received a gastrostomy or surgical implantation of a feeding tube directly through the abdominal wall into her stomach. In one week in April of 1984, Mrs. Hier pulled the gastrostomy tube from her abdomen on several occasions. She was transferred from the nursing home to a local hospital, where it was determined that surgical reinsertion was necessary. She refused the reinsertion and, in addition, resisted the administration of Thorazine. A petition was filed with a local probate court for appointment of a guardian with authority to consent to the administration of Thorazine and to surgery that would enable adequate nutritional support. Subsequent to initiating the action, the petitioners revised their position, still advocating the administration of Thorazine but, in accordance with the recommendation of physicians, opposing any surgical intervention. The probate judge authorized the administration of Thorazine but not the surgery to replace the feeding tube. The Massachusetts Appeals Court offered support for the decision of the probate judge.

Two physicians who evaluated Mrs. Hier recommended against surgery. One did so because of the patient's apparent refusal to have tube feedings. The other recommended against surgery because he thought enough resources had already been expended on the patient:

> [We] are also dealing with a patient that is requiring an enormous amount of professional time both medically and legally. . . . I now feel that enough time has been given to this patient that these efforts could be better directed towards other endeavors. . . . There comes a time when it is economically untenable to proceed with this type of treatment and it has become inordinately expensive in this situation. [Annas, 1984, p. 25]

Neither of these physicians mentioned the inevitable outcome of not performing surgery: Mrs. Hier would die of starvation if she were not fed. One physician treated the patient as a competent adult who, in the state of Massachusetts, has a right to reject medical treatment that is accorded by law of consent. The second treated Mrs. Hier as a resource allocation problem. This second view would seem the more ominous, for it appears to support the delusion that if *cure* is not possible, then there is little point to continued *care* (Meilaender, 1984).

Why did the courts assent to the approach represented by these physicians? First, as George Annas (1984) rightly observes, the courts seemed to find Mary Hier suffering from two conditions: chronic mental illness and an aversion to feeding tubes. The court ordered an appropriate medical treatment for one but rejected intervention for the other, ignoring the issue of whether or not providing nourishment is a medical treatment. Food and drink provide a nourishment that sustains all human beings, whether healthy or ill. To withdraw the nourishment is to take a direct action the only result of which can be death (Meilaender, 1984). Though neither Probate nor Appeals Court explicitly dealt with the relationship between the two conditions, the Appeals Court at least implies its recognition of such a relationship in its concluding paragraph, observing the "possibility that the Thorazine treatment authorized by the judge may, by lessening Mrs. Hier's agitation, cause her to become acquiescent towards the surgery." Further, both courts failed to heed an examining psychiatrist who testified that administration of the Thorazine through a feeding tube would be safer and less painful than administration by hypodermic needle, thus ignoring the possibility that a single surgical procedure might have permitted the patient to be fed and medicated.

Second, and perhaps more important, the Appeals Court in this case has used the substituted-judgment doctrine to create the impression of supporting the rights of mentally ill aged persons. The substituted-judgment standard, originally constructed in the Saikewicz case in Massachusetts (370 N.E. 2d 417, Mass. App., 1977), has been employed to protect incompetent patients who have never been able to express their preferences competently. Let me quote the Appeals Court in Mary Hier's case:

> Mrs. Hier's repeated dislodgments of gastric tubes, her resistance to attempts to insert a nasogastric tube, and her opposition to surgery all may be seen as a plea for privacy and personal dignity by a ninety-two-year-old person who is seriously ill and for whom life has little left to offer. [*In re* Mary Hier, 464 N.E. 2d 965, Mass. App. 1984]

Rather than treating Mary Hier as an incompetent mentally ill patient who has never been able to express her preferences competently, the court here treats Mrs. Hier as a competent patient experiencing an agonizing death. Rather than protecting the rights of incompetent elderly, the court seems to be making a significant statement about the resources that should be expended on aged, mentally ill patients in nursing homes. In effect, the Hier court reads the Saikewicz case as saying that we do not have to give older mentally retarded patients access to chemotherapy treatments because they won't understand the treatments. It reads the Earle Spring case (Kart, 1981) as saying that we do not have to give nursing home patients access to dialysis if they don't like it. And, by its own ruling, the court says that we do not have to feed mentally ill nursing home patients who pull out their feeding tubes because they don't want to be fed in that fashion.

Finally, the courts neglected entirely the sentiment and symbolism tied up with food and feeding in our society. According to psychoanalyst Erik Erikson (1968), the first sustained human contact is the mother-infant relationship in which infant trust of the mother is learned as a function of the interaction associated with the feeding process. The courts have failed to consider the possibility that denying food to a patient will increase the patient's emotional as well as physical suffering—and, perhaps, the suffering of family members and even members of the broader community. As one writer puts it, "If there is any way in which the living can stand by those who are not yet dead, it would seem to be through the provision of food and drink even when the struggle against disease has been lost" (Meilaender, 1984, p. 13).

## SUMMARY AND CONCLUSION

A significant proportion of elderly Americans remain nutritionally vulnerable. A wide array of social, cultural, and economic factors affect food intake and the nutritional status of the elderly. Income is a primary factor in determining diet at all ages. In fact, gerontologists believe the major problem in geriatric nutrition is a function not of age but rather of the income status of the aged. Impoverished elderly and those at risk of impoverishment make numerous nutritional adjustments, quite like the adjustments made by the poor of all ages.

A popular political ideology views federal involvement in social and health programs in negative terms. Four additional reasons contribute to the absence of any national nutrition policy initiative that might be of advantage to the elderly (among a wide array of interested constituent groups who would benefit from a federal nutrition policy). These include the following: (1) nutrition has been and continues to be a low federal priority item; (2) the federal government seems to associate nutrition with "income maintenance" programs; (3) the quality of the government's information on the relationship among nutrition, health, and disease is poor; and (4) it is difficult to achieve agreement among nutrition experts about public policy issues.

The medical-legal environment seems also to contain negative implications for the nutritional status of especially vulnerable older people. Heretofore, feeding and hydration have *not* been defined as scarce medical resources in this society. In the court case of Mary Hier, a Massachusetts Appeals Court has established a legal precedent that indicates the acceptability of denying food and water to an aged, mentally ill nursing home patient. If food and water become defined as scarce medical resources, like chemotherapy and hemodialysis, for example, literally thousands of nursing home patients as well as many elderly living homebound in the community run the risk of being denied access to them.

# 7

# Food and Drug Fads among the Elderly

*Linda A. Hershey*

The elderly are more exposed than other age groups to advertising from radio, television, newspapers, and magazines. They often fall prey to promoters of "health foods" of dubious value and possible risk ( Rivlin, 1983). The House of Representatives' Select Committee on Aging recently reported that many older people are so lonely that they welcome a friendly face at the door or a friendly voice on the telephone. They are prime targets for food and drug fads that play on their fears of becoming sick and helpless (Eastman, 1984).

Patients with chronic diseases such as arthritis and cancer are especially susceptible to promises of a "quick fix." Thirteen percent of the patients interviewed in one major cancer center had used or were using an additional unorthodox regimen (Cassileth, Lusk, Strouse, & Bodenheimer, 1984). The three most common unorthodox treatments included metabolic therapy, diet therapies, and megadoses of vitamins. Although some unorthodox practitioners fit the characteristic portrait of quacks and charlatans, most (60%) were physicians, few charged high fees, and most sincerely believed in the efficacy of their treatments. Patients with more education or higher social status were not automatically invulnerable. In fact, Cassileth et al.'s (1984) study showed that cancer patients receiving unorthodox treatment with or without conventional therapy were more likely to be white and better educated than those on conventional therapy alone.

## METABOLIC THERAPY

Metabolic therapy is based on the theory that toxins and waste materials in the body interfere with metabolism and healing. Metabolic regimens may include special dietary additives or chronic cleansing with various enemas. Mechnikov (1908), a respected scientist at the turn of the century, was one of the first to popularize the idea that health problems were at least partially due to intestinal putrefaction. He theorized that toxins produced by microorganisms in the gastrointestinal tract could be absorbed into the body and thereby cause disease. In his book, *Prolongation of Life* (Mechnikov, 1908), he proposed prevention of premature aging by combating the poisons with "good" bacteria that would crowd out the others. The winning candidate for his intestinal "Mr. Clean" was *Lactobacillus bulgaricus*, which had to be administered in sour milk. Why was the Slavic saprophyte chosen? Mechnikov's own epidemiologic investigation of the geographic distribution of centenarians revealed that Bulgarian peasants were outstanding in their longevity. We still see this alluded to on our television screens: Balkans eating yogurt and (therefore?) living to a ripe old age.

## DIET THERAPY

Diet therapy has a long history based on the exaggerated belief in the effects of nutrition on health and disease (Jarvis, 1983). The macrobiotic diet, based on Eastern yin-yang philosophical principles, is used by a majority of cancer patients who choose diet therapy (Cassileth et al., 1984). In this diet, foods and chemicals are placed on a continuum, beginning here with the most *yang* and ending with the most *yin*: meat, eggs, fish, grains, vegetables, fruits, dairy products, sugar, alcohol, drugs, and chemicals (Newmark & Williamson, 1983). Items on the extremes of this continuum are to be avoided. There are several levels of this diet, progressing step by step toward harmony of mind and body. Unfortunately, the "highest" level (brown rice alone) is the deadliest. Vitamin C deficiency, anemia, hypocalcemia, hypoproteinemia, and decreased renal function have developed in individuals following this regimen. The reason the macrobiotic diet has been popularized for cancer patients is its use of miso, a product of soybean fermentation believed to have anticancer properties (Esko, 1981).

The principle of diet therapy ("You are what you eat") has been used in promoting such far-ranging food additives as cod liver oil and "honeygar." For example, *Arthritis and Common Sense* (Alexander, 1950) was an amazingly successful book written by a layman who had a simple hypothesis. He proposed that the human body was like an automobile: It needed oil to run properly. If you had bursitis, the bursae must be dried out. If you had muscle pain, it must be because of lack of oil. How did you run out of oil? Inadequate diet. How did you fill the crankcase? Cod liver oil. How did you know if you had arthritis? Just about any symptom would qualify. So, according to Alexander's theory, if you had dry skin, dandruff, too much ear wax, too little ear wax, ridges on your nails, skin wrinkles, or buzzing in the ears, among other things, you were probably susceptible to arthritis. Everyone seemed to be a candidate for Alexander's oil! Ironically, recent studies suggest that cod liver oil may have a substantial effect in preventing atherosclerosis (Fisher et al., 1985).

Another very successful book, *Folk Medicine,* was written by a Vermont physician who also had a simple prescription for health maintenance: two teaspoons each of honey and vinegar in a glass of water (Jarvis, 1958). "Honeygar" could be taken one or more times daily, depending on how much physical and mental work one hoped to accomplish that day. The trouble began when the FDA started seizing commercially prepared honeygar because there were not adequate directions on the label for treating the nearly 50 diseases and other conditions that honeygar was intended to "cure." But Dr. Jarvis never made money from selling the honeygar—only from selling his book.

The honey and vinegar "remedy" actually dates back to the time of Hippocrates. Honey is derived from the nectar of flowering plants, which the honeybee collects. The bee supplies the invertase enzyme that converts sucrose (sugar) to glucose and fructose. Honey is not less calorigenic than sugar, although it is sweeter and thus might be consumed in smaller amounts. Honey is still thought by many people to be better than ordinary sugar. From the standpoint of safety, however, sugar should be considered superior (honey can be contaminated with botulinum toxin).

Other ancient customs reflect magical thinking about food, including the ritual of eating the hearts of stronger animals in order to acquire strength and courage. Soldiers in Madagascar shunned the meat of the hedgehog because of that animal's propensity to coil up into a ball when alarmed. This conjured up visions of cowardice unfitting for men of war (Frazer, 1951). The seemingly magical healing power of foods in curing certain deficiency diseases led to an exaggeration about the clinical efficacy of vitamins that persists even to this day (Jarvis, 1983). The French explorer Cartier observed the dramatic effects of a vitamin-C-containing extract on sailors with scurvy and recorded in his log that it cured not only the men's scurvy but "all of the diseases they ever had" (Lowenberg, Todhunter, Wilson, Feeney, & Savage, 1968, p. 15).

Many food fads have focused on the alleged harmful effects of certain foods. Centuries ago, Galen mentioned that fruits may cause fevers, arguing that his father (who was over 100) owed his longevity to never having eaten fruits. The tomato, in particular, has been maligned significantly during its lifetime. In early America it was thought to be poisonous. In early Europe it was considered an aphrodisiac. More recently, it has developed a reputation as a carcinogen. The poor tomato! The oldest "food hate" system of consequence is vegetarianism. In the Bible, Daniel requested permission from the Chief of the Court of Nebuchadnezzar for his men to be excused from the delicacies of the King's table and to be permitted to live on vegetables and water. At the end of 10 days, Daniel's units looked better than those who had been partaking of the King's food. Among the first modern American advocates of vegetarianism was Sylvester Graham of Connecticut, the father of the graham cracker. He believed that spices caused madness, that tea induced delirium tremens, and that meat inflamed the "basest" of human propensities. Unlike most of his fellow vegetarians, Graham died at the early age of 57. Nevertheless, the graham cracker has survived the Connecticut vegetarian for over a century.

Many famous people were vegetarians: Tolstoy, George Bernard Shaw, Horace Greeley, Ghandi, and Shelley. Perhaps the most dynamic of the twentieth-century carrot-crunchers was Bernard McFadden. He was a diminutive man who parlayed physical culture, vegetables, and sex into a multimillion-dollar enterprise. His traveling health show, his books, and especially his magazine (*True Story*) eventually earned millions. He converted many to a diet of whole-wheat bread, pea soup, nuts, carrot strips, fruit juice, and milk. He also encouraged sunbathing, exercise, a vigorous sex life, and complete abstinence from steak, alcohol, and the medical profession. He was both paranoid and ruthless. Even though this was a wild eccentric and an unsuccessful political candidate (senator, governor, and president!), he managed to father nine children by four wives, to parachute out of a plane on his eightieth birthday, and to make America health conscious. He died at 87, far short of the 125 years that he had planned, but enviably long for his day.

## MEGAVITAMIN THERAPY

Megavitamin therapy is the third most common unorthodox treatment chosen by cancer patients (Cassileth et al., 1984). It is based on the belief that high-dose vitamins strengthen the body's capacity to destroy malignant cells (Berkley, 1978; Newbold, 1979). Megadoses of vitamin C are rarely harmful, except in patients with the iron overload of hemochromatosis. Mixtures of ascorbic acid (vitamin C) and iron salts can generate free oxygen radicals and accelerate tissue damage ("Metal Chelation Therapy," 1985). Free radical formation is thought to be one mechanism of carcinogenesis. For example, asbestos is said to accelerate free radical formation, probably because it contains iron salts. This has been proposed as one mechanism whereby asbestos produces inflammation and cancer.

## DRUG THERAPY

Are elderly patients in America overdrugged? Even though the geriatric population represents only 11% of the total U.S. population, they account for 25 to 30% of health care expenditures in this country (Ouslander, 1981). Because drug therapy accounts for a significant portion of many elderly patients' budget and because they are at greater risk for adverse drug reactions, attention should be paid to age-related changes in drug metabolism, renal clearance, and drug sensitivity (Reidenberg, 1982). Hepatic metabolism is generally slower than average in the elderly, so lower doses of metabolized drugs are required. Renal function is often impaired, so lower doses of renally cleared drugs are needed. The aging nervous system is more sensitive to the depressant effects of benzodiazepines, so lower doses of these drugs should be administered to the elderly. By understanding and allowing for these dosing differences, prescribing for the elderly can be made safe and effective.

Physicians are as guilty of overprescribing drugs as their elderly patients are of seeking multiple therapies. In one Canadian study, 77 nursing home patients who had no obvious need for their diuretics were randomly assigned to take a placebo for a year or to continue with the diuretics (Myers, Weingert, Fisher, Gryfe, & Shulman, 1982). The frequency of heart failure or hypertension during the year did not differ significantly between the two groups. In fact, those assigned to placebo showed overall improvement in tests of renal function, serum potassium, cholesterol, and triglyceride levels.

The elderly are as vulnerable to drug fads as they are to food fads. Consider, for example, chelation therapy (intravenous infusions of EDTA), which is being used for the treatment of atherosclerosis (Bruni, 1985). EDTA is a drug approved by the FDA for the treatment of lead poisoning, acute hypercalcemia, and intoxication with other heavy metals. The effectiveness of this agent in prevention of myocardial infarction or stroke has never been demonstrated in controlled clinical trials. Nevertheless, about 250,000 patients have already been treated with EDTA infusions, and the number of "chelationists" in this country is increasing (The American Academy of Medical Preventics now represents 1,000 practitioners). This treatment takes its toll, not only in terms of adverse drug effects but also in the patient's pocketbook: A full course of therapy for one patient costs $3,000 to $6,000 per patient, none of which is reimbursable by medical insurance.

## CONCLUSIONS

Are elderly patients in the United States undernourished or overnourished? Certainly at least part of our elderly population is badly nourished. They are often poor, often lonely, and sometimes depressed. They may have bad teeth and bad eyesight and their taste buds may not be as acute as in youth. The intake of B vitamins and folate is generally adequate in the elderly population as a whole, but abuse of alcohol constitutes the single greatest cause of deficiency of these vitamins in older age groups (Rivlin, 1983). The elderly eat less calcium than they should, and they don't get out into the sun as much. It is encouraging to know that elderly women with osteoporosis can increase their bone density within six months by using a calcium-rich diet, together with calcium supplementation (Rivlin, 1983).

While a balanced diet can meet the nutritional needs of most older Americans, some individuals may definitely benefit from the use of specific supplements. Unfortunately, some nutritional supplements and dietary regimens have been promoted as having preventive or curative values, even though there are no adequate data to support the claims. The same can be said for some unorthodox drug treatment programs. Clearly, more research is needed in studying the nutritional problems of the elderly and in developing safer drugs to meet their special needs.

Finally, we should do more to inform our patients and the public at large about nutrition and drugs. Education is, after all, the best hope in the struggle against misinformation (Jarvis, 1983).

# Part III
# Introduction to Drug-Nutrition Interaction

# Introduction

This final section of the text addresses the difficult task of bringing together the two complex and as yet incompletely understood fields of pharmacology and nutrition as they interact in the care of the elderly patient. In the following section, five authors take a look at these fields from different viewpoints, ranging from that of the clinical investigator to the practical and applied discipline of nursing.

In Chapter 8, Shock sets the stage for this section by reviewing age decrements in performance, noting individual as well as organ system differences in the effects of aging. Aging is a normal part of the life cycle and is associated with a slowing of responses and a reduction in reserve capacities, which increase susceptibility to diseases. He highlights the problems of drugs, such as side effects, polypharmacy, and compliance, and he discusses the potential role of nutrition in the prevention and treatment of specific diseases such as hypertension, osteoporosis, and cardiovascular disease. This overview of age-related issues of drug and nutrition interaction ends with a discussion of the individual's rights and responsibilities for maintaining health and receiving treatment.

Anderson, in Chapter 9, describes drug-nutrient interrelationships as manifested in controlled clinical trials of regulated diet in young experimental subjects. Extrapolating these results to similar problems in the elderly, he suggests that age-related changes in drug metabolism, specifically in pharmacokinetics and pharmacodynamics, may in part be the result of changes in diet with age. Whether or not this proves to be the case, these studies suggest that, at the very least, clinical geriatricians need to begin to think about smoking, protein, and the consumption of such foods as cabbage and charcoal-broiled meat when prescribing drugs that are detoxified in the liver.

In Chapter 10, Chernoff takes up the practical and neglected topic of maintaining nutrition in the face of the potent side effects of cancer chemotherapy. She provides practical, experience-based guidelines for nutritional assessment of elderly cancer patients and approaches to circumventing such problems as nausea, vomiting, and anorexia. She suggests avenues by which nurses and doctors can approach their patients in a constructive, therapeutic mode and thus begin to overcome some of the neglect and aversion to which these patients are too often exposed. The recommendation of enteral nutrition when oral intake is inadequate makes sense nutritionally, but this procedure is in fact one of the earliest types of life-support system, about which so many ethical questions are currently being raised. In a situation of predictably limited duration, this approach certainly is reasonable, but it may be questioned in the case of the patient who is clearly dying.

The chapter by Whall and Booth addresses the problem of nutrition and polypharmacy in the institutionalized elderly individual. It gives some specific illustrations of the general principles of how to deal with the problem of polypharmacy as described previously in Chapter 2. Clearly, this is an issue that needs to be addressed by both the physicians who prescribe the drugs and the nurses who are required to administer them. More emphasis might indeed be put on the need for improved nurse-physician communication around such issues in the nursing home. Improved medical and nursing practice seems called for, and this must stem from more attention to these matters in primary and continuing professional education.

Finally, in Chapter 12, Dunbar re-emphasizes, again from the nursing perspective, the now-familiar problem of noncompliance and gives some sound empirical advice about how to minimize these problems in the management of the ambulatory patient.

Thus the book concludes, probably appropriately, with some glimpses of the everyday struggle in which doctors, nurses, and others are engaged as they try to use a complex array of therapeutic dietary and drug regimens for the benefit of a group of patients who, because of their age and concomitant disease, present increasingly complicated nutritional problems.

**A.B.F.**

# 8
# The Physical Functioning of the Aged

*Nathan W. Shock*

Aging is a normal part of the life cycle that affects everyone in the population in some way or another; thus, aging is not a disease in itself. Changes occur in various organs, tissues, and cells, with a net result that both physiological and psychological performances are less effective in the old than the young. In other words, aging is usually associated with some decrement in performance.

The age decrements in performance usually appear as a slowing of adaptive responses. This slowing of responses ranges from lengthening of reaction time (Surwillo & Quilter, 1964) to reductions in the rate at which new cellular enzymes can be formed within specific tissues (Barrows & Kokkonen, 1984). The general physiological basis for this slowing of responses lies in gradual reduction in the sensitivity of the physiological system involved in detecting displacements and a reduced capacity to readjust the displacement, which is often a result of the loss of functioning cells with advancing age. The older individual requires more time to decide whether or not a stimulus requires a physiological response or whether it is simply part of the "noise" in the system. Older people require more time to organize sensory inputs than do the young. For example, older automobile drivers often have difficulty in sorting out the information presented to them in an array of signs at a traffic interchange, so that they may be well through the intersection before they have observed and reacted appropriately to the information presented. Older people simply require more time to respond and adjust to displacements than the young. It is important to note, however, that, given sufficient time, older people are quite successful in making appropriate adjustments.

There are marked individual differences in the effects of aging. For example, our studies on kidney function showed that some of our 80-year-old subjects maintained a blood flow to their kidneys that was as good as the average of other individuals who were 20 years their juniors (Davies & Shock, 1950; Shock, 1952). Thus aging is influenced by many environmental factors as well as the intrinsic characteristics of each individual. It is also true that differences between individuals increase with advancing age. A group of 20-year-old subjects is much more homogeneous with respect to most performances than is a group of 60- or 70-year-old subjects.

The rate of aging varies among different organ systems. Some physiological characteristics such as fasting blood sugar levels or the acidity of the blood do not change with age; however, most functions show gradual reductions in performance. Average decrements between the ages of 30 and 80 years range from 10% (basal oxygen consumption) to 60% (maximum breathing capacity) (Shock, 1962).

Aging does not progress at the same rate in different organ systems, even within the same individual (Shock, 1962). Thus, a 60-year-old subject may have the cardiac output that is equivalent to the average for 60-year-olds, but his kidney function may be as good as that of the average 50-year-old. Observations from the Baltimore Longitudinal Study of Aging (BLSA) show that individuals vary widely in rates and pathways of aging. Although the average pathway of aging of the kidney shows a downward trend (Shock, 1952), individual subjects vary widely with respect to the rate of fall and some subjects actually show improvement in function, even in adult life (Lindeman, Tobin, & Shock, 1984). Thus, longitudinal observations that trace the pathways of aging in individual subjects emphasize the individualistic nature of aging. It is clear that there is no single aging process, nor is there good evidence that there is any single organ system or group of cells in the body that regulate the overall rate of aging for an individual. This finding has important implications for devising methods for intervening in altering rates of aging. If interventions are to be successful they must be focused on deficiencies in specific organs or cells, as there is no evidence that a single treatment or pill can alter all aging processes within an individual.

The effects of aging are more marked in performances that require the coordinated activity of different systems than in simple performances. For example, the maximum rate at which subjects can turn a crank begins to fall by age 40. In contrast, the maximum static force that can be generated by the same muscles that are involved in turning the crank is well maintained until age 60 or 65. The crank turning, which requires the coordinated activity of different muscle groups through the integrated activity of the nervous and muscular systems, shows the effect of aging before the strength of contraction of individual muscles shows any impairment (Shock & Norris, 1970). Aging is associated with a breakdown of many integrating mechanisms (Shock, 1977).

It also has been shown that aging affects well-practiced performance less than performances that are carried out only occasionally. Practice and use maintain functions that may otherwise deteriorate with aging. Thus, some impaired performances seen in older people may be due to atrophy from disuse and therefore may be avoided by maintaining physical and mental activities.

This volume has examined in some detail the potential effects of drugs, nutrition, and lifestyles on aging. In view of the central position of disease in producing disability among older people, the use of drugs among them has been analyzed. Polypharmacy is a pressing problem in dealing with the elderly. Their multiple complaints make them easy targets for multiple medications. Furthermore, they may see a number of different physicians, each of whom may prescribe a drug for a specific complaint, without regard to other drugs the patient may be receiving. Studies have found that old people are, on the average, taking at least 3 drugs, and some may be taking as many as

11 (Kart & Metress, 1984). The importance of minimizing the number of drugs prescribed for older patients and the need for periodic review of drugs being taken by each patient is a central theme of this book.

Old people are vulnerable to unique hazards from the side effects of drugs. Drugs may have special effects in old subjects because of physiological changes with aging, such as impaired absorption or changes in body composition that may affect tissue concentration of administered drugs. The physiological age reduction in kidney function observed in old subjects reduces the rate of elimination of some drugs from the body, so that exposure to the drug may be prolonged.

Compliance is also a major problem in the use of drugs in treating older subjects. Memories are often short. Schedules may not be followed, so wide variations in drug dosages may occur. The basic requirements in the drug treatment of elderly patients are (1) to keep the number of drugs to a minimum and (2) to keep the administration schedule simple.

The important role of nutrition in the prevention and treatment of specific diseases needs to be emphasized. Coronary artery disease, hypertension, osteoporosis, and diabetes respond to some degree to diet therapy. There has been a recent reemphasis on the importance of dietary fat and blood cholesterol levels in influencing the development of coronary artery disease. Although the definitive epidemiological study relating cholesterol and dietary fat to coronary artery disease has not been done, the presumptive evidence of an association is very strong for people with lifetime dietary habits related to fat intake. High fat intake and high blood cholesterol levels *do* represent risk factors for the development of coronary artery disease.

Another dietary factor that can influence the development of a disease state is salt. Many clinical studies have now shown that in many patients suffering from hypertension, blood pressure falls when salt intake is reduced. In some patients hypertension can be controlled by reducing salt intake. McCarron and his colleagues (McCarron, Morris, Henry, & Stanton, 1984) have reanalyzed measures of health and nutrition obtained from interviews and examinations of 10,372 persons (U.S. Department of Health, Education and Welfare, 1977) aged 18 to

74 years. These observations were correlated with measurements of blood pressure (McCarron et al., 1984). The analysis showed that hypertensive subjects consumed *less* sodium than those with normal blood pressure and significantly less calcium, potassium, vitamin A, and vitamin C. The meaning of these findings is not yet clear, but the idea that a lack of calcium rather than an excess of sodium may cause high blood pressure is new and deserves further exploration. It is obvious that much remains to be learned about the relationship between nutrition and disease.

Another condition that affects elderly people, especially women, is osteoporosis. Although studies on rats indicate a gradual loss of calcium with advancing age, similar loss observed in humans is usually regarded as a reflection of disease. Reanalysis of findings based on metabolic balance data collected over the past decade has led to the conclusion that daily calcium intake in adults should be about 1,000 mg/day, rather than the 600–800 mg/day now recommended.

Gross obesity remains as a risk factor for cardiovascular disease, diabetes, and breakage of bones and joints subjected to excess weight. However, reanalysis of data on the relationship between body weight and mortality rates indicates clearly that the Metropolitan Life Insurance tables of ideal weight for given body height (and build), which have been used so extensively in the United States to judge relative degrees of obesity, specify body weights that are too low. New standards have been proposed that relate body weight to minimum mortality rates. In general, optimal body weights are about 10% higher than the values given in the original Metropolitan tables (Andres, 1985). Plumpness, yes; fatness, no.

Unfortunately, it is not possible to specify with any degree of precision the optimal nutritional requirements for humans. Metabolic balance studies in humans are not apt to yield an answer, even if carried out. This is because of the great adaptability of the human animal. Agreement is needed on the criterion by which optimal adult nutrition is judged. Growth rate, which served nutritionists and physiologists so well in setting nutritional requirements for optimal growth, will no longer serve. Mortality rates may be the answer.

In addition to the physiological aspects of nutrition, the psychological and social aspects of nutritional programs for the aged need to be stressed. The giving and sharing of food have important psychological connotations in showing that someone cares for an individual. Thus food programs may serve as the central focus around which other programs providing services to old people may be organized. Food can serve as the magnet that draws older people into social programs and thus reduces the isolation experienced by many older people. The values of nutrition programs for the elderly may extend well beyond the physiological effects of food alone.

Ethical issues involved in the rights of individuals to refuse treatment are also a factor in nutrition. Few people are willing to consider alternatives to the current philosophy prevalent in law, medicine, and theology that life, even if only a vegetative existence, must be preserved at all costs, without regard to the wishes of the patient. As medical technology improves, the capability to maintain life may far outstrip our ability to arrive at ethically acceptable decisions about when artificial supports to life should be applied and how long they should be continued. In our society, with its concern for human rights, the right to die assumes increasing importance as the ultimate right of an individual.

Lifestyles also determine rates of aging. The major aspects of lifestyles that affect aging include cigarette smoking and the maintenance of physical and mental activity. Many studies have identified deleterious effects of cigarette smoking on such pulmonary functions as vital capacity and maximum breathing capacity. Smokers at all ages show poorer performance in all of these functions than do nonsmokers. When cigarette smokers stop smoking, the depressed pulmonary functions return to normal values within 12 to 18 months (Edelman, Mittman, Norris, Cohen, & Shock, 1966). It has become clear that smoking contributes to the risk of developing pulmonary disease, including lung cancer. The incidence of coronary artery disease is also greater among smokers than among nonsmokers. All evidence points to the conclusion that cigarette smoking is bad for health and longevity, although many of the deleterious effects are reversed when cigarette smoking is stopped.

The maintenance of physical and mental activity is a major factor in maintaining health and vigor to the elderly. Participation in meaningful community activities has a positive effect on health status. The role of physical activity in maintaining health and reducing the probability of developing coronary artery disease is still controversial. Although many studies report that subjects who participate in regular programs of exercise feel better, objective physiological evidence of improvement in health status is questionable. Nevertheless, subjects who regularly participate in exercise programs are in better physical condition, as measured by rate of recovery of oxygen consumption, respiratory volume, blood pressure, and heart rate after exercise, than are those who do not. Achievement of beneficial results requires a regular exercise program of 20 to 30 minutes at least three days per week. Strenuous exercise is not required. In fact, running and jogging may be ill advised among elderly subjects. Moderation is the key word for aging people.

The primary aspects of lifestyles that play a role in healthy aging include (1) refraining from smoking; (2) adjusting nutrition to activity level in order to maintain a stable body weight and to avoid gross obesity; (3) consuming a varied diet in order to assure an adequate intake of vitamins and minerals; (4) avoiding drugs which should be taken only when clearly indicated, on the advice of a physician; and (5) maintaining physical and mental activity. Longer life is within our grasp.

# 9

# Drug-Nutrient Interrelationships and the Elderly

*Karl E. Anderson*

A variety of chemicals, including drugs, environmental pollutants, and endogenous substances such as steroid hormones, are extensively metabolized in the liver prior to their excretion from the body. Two major enzyme systems are primarily responsible for these metabolic transformations. The first is termed the *mixed function oxidase system* and is found primarily in the endoplasmic reticulum of the liver and certain other tissues such as the intestine. This inducible enzyme system catalyzes the oxidation of a wide variety of chemical substrates (Conney, 1967). Cytochrome P-450, which is a family of hemoproteins in the endoplasmic reticulum, serves as the terminal oxidase for this system (Coon, 1978). The second system consists of *conjugating enzymes*, which are localized in the endoplasmic reticulum or the cytoplasm and form glucuronides, sulfates, glutathione conjugates, and other conjugates. Many oxidized products

The studies summarized here were carried out in collaboration with a number of other investigators, including A. Kappas, J. Schneider, J. Fishman, and H. L. Bradlow at The Rockefeller University Hospital, New York, NY; and A. H. Conney, E. J. Pantuck, and C. B. Pantuck, Hoffman-LaRoche, Inc., Nutley, NJ. Their contributions are gratefully acknowledged.

of the mixed-function oxidase system are substrates for these conjugating enzymes.

It has been known for some time that foods can interact directly with drugs in the gastrointestinal tract of animals as well as humans. Such direct drug-nutrient interactions may either delay or enhance drug absorption (Roe, 1978). There is also an extensive literature showing that nutrition can influence chemical transformations of drugs and other foreign substances in the liver and intestine of laboratory animals (Campbell & Hayes, 1974; Pantuck, Hsiao, Kuntzman, & Conney, 1975; Wade, Norred, & Evans, 1978; Wattenberg, 1971). However, the effects of dietary alterations on the postabsorptive metabolism of drugs in humans have been studied only recently. The purpose of this chapter is to summarize these studies, which have been carried out primarily in young, normal subjects at The Rockefeller University Hospital by the author and colleagues, and to draw attention to possible important implications for the elderly.

Recently we also have shown that dietary factors can substantially influence the metabolism of both androgens and estrogens in humans (Anderson, Kappas, Conney, Bradlow, & Fishman, 1984; Kappas et al., 1983). Dietary effects on the metabolic transformations of steroid hormones have been the subject of very few prior studies in animals or humans and are potentially important to the elderly. The frequency of neoplasms in steroid-hormone-responsive tissues, such as breast, endometrium, and prostate, increases with age, and sex steroid hormones and certain of their active metabolites have a potential role in the genesis of these and perhaps other diseases.

## MACRONUTRIENT EFFECTS ON DRUG AND STEROID HORMONE METABOLISM

The effects of the isocaloric substitution of dietary protein for either carbohydrate or fat on the metabolism of antipyrine and theophylline have been studied in normal male subjects (Alvares, Anderson, Conney, & Kappas, 1976; Anderson, Conney, & Kappas, 1979, 1982; Kappas, Anderson, Conney, & Alvares,

1976). Antipyrine and theophylline have been used by a number of investigators to assess the mixed-function oxidase system *in vivo* (Anderson et al., 1982; Davies & Thorgeirsson, 1971; Lindgren, Collste, Norlander, & Sjöqvist, 1974; Miller, Slusher, & Vesell, 1985; Vesell, 1979a; Vestal et al., 1975). They are rapidly absorbed when given by mouth to fasting subjects, and their metabolic clearance rates reflect the activities of one or more species of hepatic cytochrome P-450. The *in vivo* transformation of antipyrine consists of 4-hydroxylation, N-demethylation, and 3-methyl-hydroxylation; while theophylline undergoes N-demethylation and 8-oxidation. The products of these oxidation reactions are then conjugated, and the conjugates are readily excreted in urine.

The subjects in these studies consumed carefully calculated test diets for consecutive two-week periods. Single doses of each drug were given on separate days during each test-diet period, and serial blood (or saliva) samples were obtained for measurement of drug concentrations. Plots of these data over time were employed to calculate plasma half-lives, apparent volumes of distribution, and metabolic clearance rates. Test diets contained calculated amounts of protein, carbohydrate, and fat and consisted mostly of weighed portions of solid foods rich in one or more of these macronutrients.

In an initial study in six normal subjects (see Table 9.1), the isocaloric change from the high-protein to the high-carbohydrate diet resulted in a decrease in dietary protein from 44% to 10% of total calories, while carbohydrate intake increased from 35% to 70%. Dietary fat remained constant at 20% to 21% of total calories. During the high protein intake, the average plasma half-lives of both drugs were shorter, and metabolic clearance rates substantially greater than during the high-carbohydrate dietary period. There were no significant changes in the apparent volumes of distribution. The results indicated that the drugs were metabolized more rapidly during the high-protein dietary period. In further studies, the addition of a pure protein supplement (100g of sodium caseinate daily for 2 weeks) to a calculated well-balanced diet in two subjects increased the metabolism of both antipyrine and theophylline, while in two other subjects a pure carbohydrate supplement (200g of sucrose

TABLE 9.1

**Antipyrine and Theophylline Clearance in Six Normal Subjects during Consumption of Two Calculated Diets High in Protein or Carbohydrate[a]**

| Diet | Diet Composition (%) | | | Antipyrine MCR | Theophylline MCR |
|------|---------|-----|--------------|---------------|-----------------|
| | Protein | Fat | Carbohydrate | | |
| | | | | $(ml \cdot min^{-1} \cdot kg^{-1})$ | |
| High protein | 44 | 21 | 35 | 0.76 ± 0.04 | 1.00 ± 0.06 |
| High carbohydrate | 10 | 20 | 70 | 0.52 ± 0.06* | 0.69 ± 0.04† |

[a]Each diet was consumed by the subjects for 2 weeks. Antipyrine metabolism was studied on day 10, and theophylline metabolism on day 14 of each dietary period. Values for metabolic clearance rate (MCR) are means ±SE; the change in diet produced significant alterations in these values (*$p < 0.01$, †$< 0.002$, paired $t$-test).

daily) produced the opposite effect (Alvares et al., 1976; Anderson et al., 1982; Kappas et al., 1976).

In a second study, also in six subjects (see Table 9.2), the metabolism of antipyrine and theophylline was studied during the sequential feeding of high-carbohydrate, high-fat, and high-protein diets (Anderson et al., 1979, 1982). The compositions of these diets permitted observations of the effects of the isocaloric substitution of fat for carbohydrate while keeping the total protein content constant at 10% of total calories, as well as observations of the substitution of dietary protein for fat while keeping carbohydrate content constant at 20% of total calories. The metabolic clearance rates of both drugs were greater during the high-protein dietary period than during the consumption of the other two test diets, and there was little or no difference in drug metabolism during the high-carbohydrate and high-fat dietary periods. These results indicated that dietary protein had a more specific influence on drug oxidation rates in humans than did carbohydrate or fat.

In a third study in nine subjects (see Table 9.3), dietary protein remained constant at 15% of total calories during three test diet periods, while the effect on drug metabolism of substi-

**TABLE 9.2**
Antipyrine and Theophylline Metabolism in Six Normal Subjects
on Three Diets Differing in Protein, Carbohydrate, and Fat Content[a]

| Diet | Diet Composition (%) | | | Antipyrine MCR | Theophylline MCR |
|---|---|---|---|---|---|
| | Protein | Fat | Carbohydrate | | |
| | | | | $(ml \cdot min^{-1} \cdot kg^{-1})$ | |
| High carbohydrate | 10 | 10 | 80 | 0.57 ± 0.02 | 0.76 ± 0.06 |
| High fat | 10 | 70 | 20 | 0.59 ± 0.02 | 0.74 ± 0.04 |
| High protein | 50 | 30 | 20 | 0.71 ± 0.05*† | 0.98 ± 0.08*s |

[a]Each diet was consumed for 2 weeks in the order shown. Antipyrine metabolism was studied on day 10, and theophylline metabolism on day 14 of each dietary period. Values for metabolic clearance rate (MCR) are means ±SE. Where indicated, values during the high-protein dietary period were significantly different from the high-carbohydrate dietary period (*$p < 0.005$) or the high-fat dietary period (†$p < 0.01$, s$p < 0.02$, paired $t$-test).

**TABLE 9.3**
Effects of Substituting Saturated and Unsaturated Fat for Dietary
Carbohydrate on Drug Metabolism in Nine Normal Subjects[a]

| Diet | Diet Composition (%) | | | Antipyrine MCR | Theophylline MCR |
|---|---|---|---|---|---|
| | Protein | Fat | Carbohydrate | | |
| | | | | $(ml \cdot min^{-1} \cdot kg^{-1})$ | |
| High unsaturated fat | 15 | 60* | 25 | 0.69 ± 0.04 | 0.95 ± 0.10 |
| High carbohydrate | 15 | 25 | 60 | 0.74 ± 0.04 | 0.91 ± 0.06 |
| High saturated fat | 15 | 60† | 25 | 0.72 ± 0.03 | 0.98 ± 0.09 |

[a]Each diet was fed for two weeks. The values (means ±S.E.) for metabolic clearance rate (MCR) were not significantly different during the three dietary periods paired $t$-test).
*In the high unsaturated fat diet, 80% of the fat was in the form of corn oil.
†In the high saturated fat diet, 80% of the fat was in the form of butter; in all other respects the two high-fat diets were identical.

tuting large amounts of either polyunsaturated fat (corn oil) or saturated fat (butter) for carbohydrate was examined in nine normal subjects (Anderson et al., 1979, 1982). As expected, these substitutions produced marked changes in plasma lipids; however, there were no significant changes in metabolism of either antipyrine or theophylline. Subsequently, Mucklow et al. (1980) have reported that exchanging saturated for unsaturated fat in the diet had no effect on the metabolism of antipyrine or debrisoquin in normal subjects. These studies suggest that the content of dietary fat and carbohydrate can influence the metabolic systems that regulate plasma lipids without significantly affecting the metabolism of at least some substrates of the mixed-function oxidase system in humans.

Steroid hormones, as well as drugs, are extensively metabolized in the liver (Anderson & Kappas, 1982; Conney, 1967; Estabrook, Martinez-Zedillo, Young, Peterson, & McCarthy, 1975). Our recent studies have shown that certain major pathways for endogenous steroid hormone metabolism can also be influenced by dietary macronutrients. Isocaloric exchanges of dietary protein and carbohydrate produced substantial changes in estrogen 2-hydroxylation but did not influence estrogen $16\alpha$-hydroxylation (Anderson et al., 1984). Both of these oxidative processes are believed to be cytochrome P-450-dependent. The results indicate that these two major oxidative pathways for endogenous estrogens are not regulated in the same manner by dietary factors. The $5\alpha$-reduction of testosterone, which is catalyzed by a microsomal reductase that is not cytochrome P-450-dependent, was influenced by the diet in a reciprocal fashion (Kappas et al., 1983). Interestingly, a number of environmental agents, such as barbiturates (Kappas, Bradlow, Bickers, & Alvares, 1977) and halogenated hydrocarbons, also have been shown to increase microsomal cytochrome P-450 while decreasing $\Delta^4$-steroid-$5\alpha$-reductase activity in the liver of experimental animals. Thus, dietary protein can have metabolic effects on certain metabolic functions of the liver that are similar to those of drugs and environmental pollutants (Kappas et al., 1983). The effects of other dietary components, including fat, on steroid hormone metabolism have not as yet been examined in humans.

# CRUCIFEROUS VEGETABLES AND DRUG METABOLISM

Cabbage and brussels sprouts contain substances that can potently induce the mixed-function oxidase system in animals (Loub, Wattenberg, & Davis, 1975; Pantuck et al., 1979). We have studied the effects of these vegetables on drug oxidations and conjugations in groups of normal subjects (Pantuck et al., 1979). In these studies we compared (1) a 10-day control diet period; (2) the same control diet for 3 more days, followed by a diet containing the cruciferous vegetables for 7 days; and (3) a return to the control diet for an additional 10 days. During the test diet period, brussels sprouts and cabbage were substituted for vegetables known not to stimulate the mixed-function oxidase system in animals. This dietary change significantly enhanced the oxidation of antipyrine and phenacetin in a group of 10 subjects. For antipyrine, we observed a 13% decrease in the mean half-life and an 11% increase in the metabolic clearance rate. For phenacetin, the average plasma concentration of the drug decreased by 34 to 67% when measured repeatedly up to 7 hours after administration, and the ratio of the mean concentration of the major oxidative metabolite, N-acetyl-p-aminophenol (APAP) to phenacetin decreased. APAP is also known as acetaminophen and is a commonly used analgesic. In our study, there was also evidence that conjugation of APAP was enhanced by the cabbage–brussels-sprouts diet. This was confirmed in a more recent study in which these vegetables were shown to enhance the glucuronidation of acetaminophen in a group of 10 normal subjects (Pantuck et al., 1984).

# CHARCOAL BROILING OF MEATS

Broiling of meats over charcoal results in the formation of polycyclic aromatic hydrocarbons similar to those found in cigarette smoke. Since drug oxidations are enhanced in smokers, presumably from exposure to such chemicals (Jenne, Nagasawa, McHugh, MacDonald & Wyse, 1975; Pantuck et al., 1974), it seemed likely that charcoal-broiled beef might accelerate drug metabolism. The effects of this method of food preparation on the metabolism of phenacetin, antipyrine, theophylline, and acetaminophen have been investigated (Anderson et al., 1983; Conney et al., 1976; Kappas et al., 1978). In these studies hamburger and steak were broiled over charcoal and fed twice daily, as part of a calculated test diet, for 4 to 5 days before the administration of single doses of these drugs to normal subjects. During control-diet periods aluminum foil was placed between the meat and the burning charcoal. The only difference between the charcoal-broiled beef diet and the control diet was in this aspect of food preparation.

During the test diet the average peak concentration of phenacetin in plasma fell substantially in a group of nine subjects with ingestion of charcoal-broiled beef, and the ratio of APAP to phenacetin was increased (Conney et al., 1976). This ability of charcoal-broiled beef to increase o-dealkylation of phenacetin is similar to those reported for cigarette smoking (Pantuck et al., 1974). Data also suggested the glucuronide conjugation of APAP is not increased by charcoal-broiled beef (Conney et al., 1976). This was substantiated recently in a study of acetaminophen metabolism in nine normal subjects using a similar study design (Anderson et al., 1983).

Antipyrine and theophylline metabolism were studied utilizing the same dietary regimen (Kappas et al., 1978). Mean plasma half-lives for both drugs were decreased by 22% and were accompanied by reciprocal increases in metabolic clearance rates when charcoal-broiled meat was consumed. Thus, food prepared in this maner can enhance the oxidation rates of several drug substrates in humans but, in contrast to cabbage and brussels sprouts, does not enhance acetaminophen conjugation (Anderson et al., 1983; Pantuck et al., 1984).

## IMPLICATIONS

The fact that diet, and specific components in the diet, can influence the metabolism of drugs and steroid hormones in humans has wide-ranging implications, many of which are relevant to the aging population. Diet-induced changes in steroid hormone metabolism, for example, could influence the genesis of neoplastic and other diseases in hormone-responsive tissues. Interindividual variations in drug metabolism rates are considerable and are important considerations in therapeutics in any age group. Such interindividual variations are determined in part by genetic factors (Miller et al., 1985; Vesell, 1979b; Vesell & Page, 1968). The environment is also an important determinant of interindividual differences in drug metabolism rates and can in addition result in variability over time in the same individuals (Alvares et al., 1979). Vesell and Page (1969) have demonstrated genetic control of the inducing effect of a barbiturate on drug (antipyrine) metabolism, which indicates that there are important interactions between inheritable factors and environmental stimuli in determining drug metabolism rates.

Age is one of many additional factors that may influence drug disposition. Several groups of investigators have reported a general decline with age in the metabolism of certain drugs in humans (Greenblatt, Sellers, & Shader, 1982; O'Malley, Crooks, Duke, & Stevenson, 1971; Triggs, Nation, Long, & Ashley, 1975; Vestal et al., 1975; Vestal, Wood, Branch, Shand, & Wilkinson, 1979). Drug conjugations appear to be less subject to the influences of age than are drug oxidations. In addition to effects on drug metabolism, changes in body composition and drug distribution, protein binding, and renal clearance can occur with aging. Decreased clearance of some drugs that are rapidly taken up by the liver may be explained by decreased hepatic blood flow in the elderly (Wood, Vestal, Wilkinson, Branch, & Shand, 1979). Metabolism rates of more slowly cleared drugs, such as antipyrine, are not dependent upon hepatic blood flow, and decreased metabolism rates of such drugs are more likely to reflect changes in the hepatic content or activity of the mixed-function oxidase system.

In laboratory animals, aging may produce changes in the enzyme components of the mixed-function oxidase system or in the membrane environment of these enzymes (Kato, 1978; Schmucker, 1985). In limited studies of human liver specimens obtained mostly by percutaneous biopsy, no age-related changes in this hepatic enzyme system have been observed *in vitro* (James, Rawlins, & Woodhouse, 1982). It remains uncertain, therefore, whether differences of *in vivo* drug metabolism rates between young and old subjects reflect an effect of aging on hepatic enzymes or changes in those environmental factors, including diet, that are known to influence the oxidation of foreign and endogenous chemicals in the liver. Changes in lifestyle and economic circumstances with age might well be associated with a decrease in the intake of certain foods, such as protein-rich foods and charcoal-broiled meats, thus contributing to age-associated changes in drug oxidation rates.

Vestal and co-workers (Vestal et al., 1975; Vestal, Wood, Branch, et al., 1979) have shown that at least one environmental factor, namely cigarette smoking, may explain part of the difference between young and old subjects in oxidation rates of drugs such as antipyrine and propranolol. This is not surprising because smoking is known to have an inducing effect on drug oxidations in younger subjects, and smokers are less likely than nonsmokers to survive to an advanced age. It is of interest that drug oxidations in elderly individuals appeared to be less responsive to the inducing effects of smoking than in younger subjects, suggesting that the inducibility of the hepatic mixed-function oxidase system might decrease with age (Wood et al., 1979). It would be of interest to compare in young and old subjects the responsiveness of the mixed-function oxidase system to dietary stimuli.

Our studies also have implications for certain types of patients in whom nutrition may be impaired. For example, in chronic liver disease a variable degree of impairment of drug metabolism has been reported, and the intake of protein and other nutrients may be reduced. Dietary histories in one such study of patients with chronic liver disease indicated that decreased protein intake was an important determinant of impaired drug metabolism (Farrell, Cooksley, Hart, & Powell, 1978). In a group of hospitalized children with asthma, Feldman and co-workers (1980) found that dietary protein could influence steady-state plasma concentrations of theophylline and the effectiveness of treatment. As reviewed elsewhere (Anderson et al., 1982), drug metabolism also may be impaired in adults and children with protein-calorie malnutrition. However, from studies of this condition it is difficult to discern which nutritional factors are most important in influencing drug metabolism rates. Drug metabolism has been reported to be unaltered following elective starvation for obesity (Reidenberg, 1977) and in anorexia nervosa (Bakke, Aanderud, Syversen, Bassoe, & Myking, 1978).

Changes in the enzyme systems that metabolize drugs, hormones, and other chemicals can alter the response of the host to such chemical exposures. It is now clear that certain specific dietary components can substantially influence these metabolic systems in humans, and it seems appropriate to consider that such nutritional influences on chemical metabolism may have important implications for the elderly.

# 10
# Nutrition and Chemotherapy in the Elderly

*Ronni Chernoff*

Cancer is a disease that primarily occurs late in life; the mean age of people who have cancer is 67.5 years (Yancik, 1983). This is related to many factors, among them (1) the length of time some cancers take to develop (e.g., those caused by environmental pollutants or cigarette smoking); (2) the failure of the immune system, which occurs with normal aging, to combat errant cells; and (3) the development of disease in people who might, in earlier eras, have died from contagious or chronic illness before cancers had time to develop. Whatever the reasons, cancer is a major disease among elderly people, who have unique needs and health problems that distinguish them from young people.

One area that may prove to be particularly problematic for elderly cancer patients is nutrition. Nutritional status may be compromised in elderly patients if they have other chronic diseases, such as diabetes, heart disease, stroke or other neurological problems, chronic obstructive pulmonary disease, liver disease, renal disease, or gastrointestinal disease. It also may be a problem for those who live on fixed incomes, have ill-fitting dentures, are housebound, or are socially isolated. The occurrence of cancer itself may add a burden to a patient that will affect nutritional status; this may be particularly devastating in an older individual who maintains borderline nutritional status when medically stable.

There are several ways in which cancer and nutrition interact. Diet may be an etiological factor in the development of cancer; certainly many food additives have been potentially identified as carcinogens (Shubik, 1979). Cancer may have either systemic or local effects that indirectly impact on the nutritional status of the host. The treatments for cancer also may have a profound influence on the nutritional status of the patient ( Donaldson & Lenon, 1979). This chapter will examine the effects of cancer on nutritional status; the effects of cancer treatments, particularly chemotherapy, on nutritional status; and some feeding alternatives that can offset potential malnutrition in elderly cancer patients.

## EFFECTS OF CANCER ON NUTRITIONAL STATUS

Cancer can impact on nutritional status in a variety of ways. The mental image often held of a cancer patient is that of a person who has severe muscle-wasting and malnutrition. Anorexia is one of the factors in the development of cachexia, a systemic effect that is often seen in cancer patients. Cachexia is a syndrome that combines loss of appetite (anorexia), weight loss, muscle wasting, early satiety, and possible alterations of energy metabolism. Anorexia has many etiologies and is not limited to cancer patients, but it may be seen in patients with other life-threatening, systemic illnesses. Despite an association with emotional factors, the effects of appetite loss and inability to eat are as important and difficult to manage as if the association were with a measurable disease process. Anorexia may occur at times of severe emotional stress, such as during the anticipation of diagnosis when the patient may suspect the worst but has not yet had it confirmed. It also may occur when the diagnosis is made, while waiting to find out what the treatment options are and what the prognosis might be, after treatment, when disease recurs or metastases are identified, and during times of pain or discomfort (Holland, Rowland, & Plumb, 1977; Smale, 1979).

The effects of anorexia are no less devastating when they are etiologically emotional than when they are physically induced. Anorexia may be a result of the treatments used for cancer, including surgery, radiation therapy, and chemotherapy (Brennan, 1979; Donaldson & Lenon, 1979; Welch, 1981). The pain and discomfort of surgery and the effects of stress, nausea, vomiting, diarrhea, esophagitis, enteritis, and other gastrointestinal distresses may contribute to a severe loss of appetite in patients treated for cancer.

Anorexia is also associated with the disease process of cancer. Sometimes, as with pancreatic cancer, weight loss associated with anorexia may be the first symptom. Anorexia is associated with cancers in the gastrointestinal tract and often is a symptom of advanced-stage cancers (Holland, Rowland, & Plumb, 1977). Whatever the etiology, the effects of anorexia, leading to cachexia, are serious and must be addressed as part of the overall treatment plan. Anorexia may be particularly dangerous in the elderly, who may have depleted nutritional stores or may have an impaired ability to overcome the stresses associated with cancer and cancer treatment.

Cancer may affect nutritional status by interfering with the ability of the patient to ingest adequate calories and nutrients (Shils, 1979). There may be mechanical interference with ingestion due to the presence of a tumor. Irritation of the oral or upper gastrointestinal mucosa may occur if these tissues or adjacent tissues are treated with radiation therapy. Mouth sores may develop as a side effect of various chemotherapeutic agents. Particularly in patients who have cancer in the head and neck or upper gastrointestinal tract, there may be great pain with chewing and swallowing. Tumors in the distal gastrointestinal tract may lead to obstructions that make eating difficult.

Treatment effects may interfere with adequate ingestion of food. Surgery on the gastrointestinal tract may render it useless for a period of time, chemotherapy may lead to gastrointestinal disturbances that interfere with normal eating, and radiation therapy may cause enteritis. Long-term effects of cancer treatment (radiation therapy or surgery) may occur because of adhesions and potential obstruction. In elderly patients, the time required to recover may be extended, since it takes longer for their systems to recover from an insult and to heal properly (Shock, 1982). Adequate nutrition is a major factor in normal healing, but normal healing requires higher levels of some nutrients, especially protein, vitamin C, and energy substrate.

Malabsorption may occur in cancer patients for several reasons. Pancreatic or biliary insufficiency may occur due to tumor interference; surgery may lead to a short bowel; radiation may damage absorptive surfaces; chemotherapy may interfere with the absorption of certain nutrients by acting as analogues; malnutrition may lead to malabsorption. Malnutrition, or the inadequate provision of essential nutrients, especially to metabolically active tissue, will contribute to an impairment of normal tissue regeneration. Since the absorptive surface of the bowel is replaced approximately every 72 to 120 hours, an inadequate intake of protein and energy substrate required to make new cells will lead to a bowel surface that has immature and therefore less-than-optimal cell functioning (Greene, 1983). The gastrointestinal tract is particularly vulnerable due to the rapid turnover of epithelial cells. Their rapid division makes them particularly vulnerable to the effects of chemotherapy (Ohnuma & Holland, 1977; Shaw, Spector, & Ladman, 1979). In the elderly, recovery may be slower and prolonged injury to the gastrointestinal tract will lead to continued malabsorption. This in turn will lead to malnutrition. Another effect of the immature bowel surface is the loss of the ability to make needed enzymes for digestion. An example of this is an induced lactase deficiency. Inadequate amounts of lactase, which cleaves lactose into its monosaccharide components (glucose and galactose), may lead to lactose intolerance. Ironically, milk, the source of lactose, is often suggested to cancer patients as a calorie-protein supplement. It would be wise to consider the use of lactose-free milk substitutes for malnourished cancer patients.

Cancer patients may lose nutrients for other reasons than malabsorption. One cause of nutrition debilitation may be protein-losing enteropathies. Protein may be lost due to obstructed gastrointestinal lymphatics, loss of exudate through inflamed mucosa, excessive mucus secretion, and excessive losses secondary to other problems such as fistulous losses, renal damage, or liver toxicity. Fluid and electrolyte problems may occur due to unusual fluid losses (Welch, 1981).

In the elderly cancer patient, fluid and electrolyte problems may be particularly troublesome. They may be related to vomiting, diarrhea, fistulous losses, renal or hepatic dysfunction, and over- or underhydration (Flombaum, Isaacs, Scheiner, & Vanamee, 1981). Many bedfast elderly have inadequate fluid intake or an impaired thirst sensation due to depressed central nervous system function (Lindeman, 1982). It is important that fluid balance be carefully monitored in cancer patients for all of these reasons.

## NUTRITIONAL SIDE EFFECTS OF CHEMOTHERAPY

The side effects of chemotherapy are well documented. Few clinicians, however, have examined the effects of chemotherapy in the elderly, choosing instead to focus on groups defined by diagnosis. There are some considerations that are unique to the elderly patient that must be mentioned. The toxic side effects of chemotherapeutic agents, shown in Table 10.1, are well known to oncologists. In the past, elderly patients with other chronic diseases requiring management with medications have not been considered candidates for intensive chemotherapy because of anticipated drug interactions. In fact, more recently it has been found that elderly patients can withstand aggressive treatment with chemotherapy with appropriate monitoring (Kerr & Chabner, 1983). One consideration, however, is the alteration of drug distribution that may occur in an elderly cancer patient. Changes in body composition, with a loss of water and lean body mass and an increase in total body fat, may reduce the volume of drug distributed throughout the body, thereby concentrating the amount of free drug available to target tissues and leading to an increase in toxicity. A similar problem may be related to hypoalbuminemia in the elderly patient who is bor-

**TABLE 10.1**
**Nutritional Side Effects of Some Common Chemotherapeutic Agents**

| Drug | Acute Nutritional Side Effects |
| --- | --- |
| Actinomycin D | Severe nausea and vomiting, mucositis, diarrhea |
| Asparaginase | Nausea and vomiting, abdominal pain |
| Bleomycin | Nausea and vomiting, mucositis |
| Busulfan | Nausea and vomiting |
| Cisplatin | Nausea and vomiting, renal damage |
| Cyclophosphamide | Nausea and vomiting, hyponatremia, anorexia |
| Cytosine Arabinoside | Nausea and vomiting, diarrhea, oral ulceration |
| Daunorubicin | Nausea and vomiting |
| Diethylstilbesterol | Nausea and vomiting, cramps, fluid retention |
| Doxorubicin | Nausea and vomiting, diarrhea |
| Fluorouracil | Nausea and vomiting, diarrhea, oral and GI ulcers |
| Floxuridine | Nausea and vomiting, diarrhea |
| Hydroxyurea | Nausea and vomiting, stomatitis, diarrhea, buccal mucosa ulcerations |
| Mechlorethamine (nitrogen mustard) | Nausea and vomiting, anorexia |
| Mercaptopurine | Vomiting, anorexia, diarrhea, abdominal pain |
| Methotrexate | Nausea and vomiting, diarrhea, stomatitis, oral ulcers |
| Mithramycin | Anorexia, nausea, diarrhea |
| Mitotane | Nausea and vomiting |
| Prednisone | Diabetes, GI tract ulceration |
| Procarbazine | Nausea and vomiting |
| Streptozotocin | Nausea and vomiting |
| Vinblastine | Nausea and vomiting, stomatitis |
| Vincristine | Severe abdominal pain, constipation |

derline malnourished. This may decrease the protein binding of drugs, allowing more free drug to contribute to overall drug toxicity (Kerr & Chabner, 1983).

When drugs that have dosages calculated on a body-weight or body-volume basis are used, changes in body composition and weight status may affect the ability of the patient to be treated with effective drug doses.

Drug toxicities may result in the compromise of function in many organ systems, including renal, hepatic, cardiac, and gastrointestinal. In elderly patients these toxicities may be particularly devastating, especially if organ function is compromised due to age effects or chronic disease. Nutritional requirements may be altered to compensate for organ systems compromise, but perhaps more important are gastrointestinal side effects from chemotherapeutic agents. Nausea, vomiting, diarrhea, constipation, abdominal pain, mucosal lesions, and mucositis will all interfere with adequate nutrient intake and maintenance of nutritional status. Fluid and electrolyte problems may develop rapidly. Patients must be closely monitored to prevent these problems from occurring and creating unnecessary untoward side effects.

Another side effect of chemotherapy may be changes in taste perception (Fong, 1979). Since loss of taste perception is a problem that has been identified in elderly people (Schiffman, 1977), the addition of chemotherapy for the treatment of cancer may seriously alter taste perceptions in elderly cancer patients. This compounds the anorexia that is related to the use of many chemotherapy agents and makes it even more difficult for elderly cancer patients to ingest adequate nutrition.

## ASSESSING NUTRITIONAL STATUS

The most direct method of monitoring the nutritional status of elderly cancer patients is to use traditional tools of nutritional assessment. There are limitations, however, to some of the measures commonly used (Chernoff, Mitchell, & Lipschitz, 1984). Many nutritional assessment measures are unreliable, and many do not have standards for individuals over age 55.

Anthropometric measures such as height, weight, skinfolds, and arm circumference are commonly used tools for evaluating changes in body composition. These measures are useful in monitoring changes in an individual over time, but they will only detect gross abnormalities that may require long periods of time to develop. Comparing individual measurements of height, weight, skinfold, or arm circumference to reference values is often invalid for an elderly patient, since commonly used standards are for young populations. In addition, stature and body composition change with age (Mitchell & Lipschitz, 1982).

One of the most obvious physical changes that occurs with aging is the decrease in stature or height. A progressive decrease in height occurs as part of the normal aging process, caused primarily by the shortening of the spinal column due to a compression of the spinal discs. Other factors that add to the decrease in height are the presence of kyphosis, severe osteoporosis, or arthritis, which may make it difficult for an afflicted individual to stand straight for an accurate measure of height. Tables that are used to determine weight-for-height standards do not compensate for changes in height with age, nor do they make adjustments for weight changes that occur as a part of the normal aging process.

Weight changes that occur with aging are partially reflective of changes in body composition. There are losses of lean body mass, fluid, and fat tissue that account for these changes. Standard tables do not reflect these alterations. Unfortunately, judgments regarding nutritional status are often made by health care practitioners who use these standard tables. Changes in weight over time for an individual, using the individual as his own control, are probably the best measures of nutritional adequacy.

Skinfold-thickness measures and arm circumference are often used to measure body composition by measuring subcutaneous fat or muscle mass. These measures are unreliable parameters of body composition in the elderly patient, due to the aforementioned changes in body composition but also to lack of standards on an aged population.

Biochemical measures that are used as part of a comprehensive nutrition assessment include serum albumin, serum transferrin, total lymphocyte count, and urinary creatinine excretion. Serum albumin and serum transferrin may be valuable measures to use as components of a thorough nutritional assessment, but it is quite important to be aware of medical reasons for changes in these values. Particularly in older patients, it is important not to confuse biochemical measures altered by the presence of cancer or by treatments used for cancer with those that indicate compromised nutritional status. The inability to maintain serum albumin levels, however, correlates with mortality in elderly cancer patients (Ching et al., 1979).

Hematological measures are often included as part of a nutritional assessment. An unexplained anemia often occurs in healthy older persons, so it is difficult to ascribe hematologic changes to nutritional status (Lipschitz, Mitchell, & Thompson, 1981). In cancer patients, anemias and depressed immunologic status occur with the disease and its treatment modalities. It is therefore difficult to ascribe these changes to nutritional status alone.

One parameter that is important to measure in elderly cancer patients is dietary intake. Accurate dietary intake documentation is a valuable record that is an obtainable, noninvasive, cost-effective measure of nutrient intake that will indicate alterations in nutrient ingestion and changes over time. Regular monitoring of dietary intake, along with periodic clinical assessments that focus on indicators of nutritional status, are the most valuable measures to use when assessing the nutritional status of elderly patients.

Patients who are at greatest risk for being or becoming malnourished are those who have chronic illnesses (diabetes, renal disease, liver disease, inflammatory bowel disease, cardiovascular disease); or who are grossly over- or underweight; have recent, rapid weight loss; severe over- or underhydration; prolonged gastrointestinal fluid losses; infection; fever; or decreased oral intake for 10 days or longer.

It is of paramount importance to monitor nutritional status regularly in elderly cancer patients. Their chemotherapeutic dose tolerance will be affected by their biochemical, hematological, and physical profiles, which may be related to their nutritional status. Patients who are in nutritional failure may be more susceptible to sepsis, delayed wound healing, poor response to therapy, and a more complicated course to recovery.

## FEEDING ELDERLY CANCER PATIENTS

Maintaining nutritional status in cancer patients requires careful, regular monitoring of nutrient intakes that begins prior to treatment. Waiting until nutritional stores are depleted and the patient has lost greater than 10% body weight will lead to a need for extraordinary measures for nutritional repletion that

**TABLE 10.2**
**Feeding Suggestions for Patients with Anorexia**

Eat small, frequent meals and snacks
Keep snacks readily available
Try untraditional meals (e.g., breakfast foods for dinner) and calorie supplements to zero-calorie liquids such as coffee or tea
Add calories whenever possible
Use flavorings or seasonings
Use variety in texture, color, and temperature

are expensive and carry health risks of their own (Chernoff, 1979). Carefully recording dietary intakes and providing supplemental foods or snacks that may be modified to meet specific patient needs may prevent or delay the use of parenteral support in cancer patients.

The most common problems that occur in cancer patients are nausea, vomiting, and anorexia. There are many dietary modifications that can be made to feed patients who are anorectic (see Table 10.2), and there are some tricks that can be used to allay nausea (see Table 10.3). However, one suggestion often made in lay literature is to use milk as a base for cooking and as a source of supplemental calories and protein (National Institutes of Health, 1979, 1980; Rosenbaum, Stitt, Drasin, & Rosenbaum, 1978, 1980). Milk is an excellent food and does add high-biological-value protein and calories; however, patients who are

**TABLE 10.3**
**Feeding Suggestions for Patients with Nausea and Vomiting**

Eat crackers or dry toast
Eat small, frequent meals
Eat slowly
Use light, dry, bland foods
Sip liquids at least 30 minutes before or after meals, to avoid gastric distention
See if cold foods may be more appealing
Eat tart or sour foods, which will help nausea if mouth sores are not present
When vomiting is present, restrict diet to sips of clear liquids

malnourished and are receiving chemotherapy or radiation therapy to the abdomen will develop, if it does not already exist, an intolerance to lactose (milk sugar). It is well known that many adults of various racial and ethnic backgrounds are lactose intolerant or lactase deficient. Providing large amounts of milk to these individuals will lead to the additional problems associated with lactose intolerance: cramping, diarrhea, bloating, flatulence, abdominal pain, and a sour taste in the mouth. Using lactose-free milk substitutes should be considered.

When modifying diets for elderly cancer patients, it is best to include the patient as part of the process; elderly patients have developed eating habits over a lifetime and cannot and will not change them simply because they are told to. The best success occurs with the least change. Nevertheless, dietary alterations should be considered when voluntary oral intake is below maintenance for the patient or when signs of malnutrition occur, such as weight loss greater than 5%, serum albumin below 3.5 g/L, or onset of gastrointestinal symptoms or stomatitis.

If modification of the oral diet is not sufficient to compensate for nutritional depletion and if weight loss continues, enteral nutrition support should be considered (Chernoff, 1979). Enteral support offers many advantages in feeding cancer patients, among them utilization of the gastrointestinal tract, nonsurgical invasion such as is necessary with parenteral nutrition, relative simplicity, and safety. Using the enteral route of feeding allows energy and protein requirements to be met; provides adequate amounts of vitamins and minerals; maintains the intestinal epithelium, which has been shown to atrophy with disuse; and allows treatment of malabsorption syndromes by permitting nutrient manipulation not possible with food or oral feedings. Enteral nutrition support in cancer patients aids in maintaining hydration status, a very important consideration in patients with fluid and electrolyte imbalances, supports weight gain, improves energy states, and maintains serum albumin by providing adequate amounts of protein substrate (Meguid, Gray, & Debonis, 1984). By maintaining weight, hydration, and serum protein integrity, enteral nutrition support contributes to the completion of cancer therapy and helps to maintain a sense of well-being for the patient.

Should enteral feeding prove a failure, the option of parenteral nutrition still exists. There is a great deal known about the
use of parenteral nutrition as an adjunct to cancer treatment
(Copeland, 1983); there is little known about special needs of
elderly patients receiving this type of nutrition (Chernoff &
Lipschitz, 1986). The parenteral nutritional support of elderly
patients is an area for future research, along with many other
questions regarding nutritional rquirements of elderly persons,
both healthy and with chronic and critical illnesses.

# 11

# Nutrition and Polypharmacy in the Institutional Care of the Elderly

*Ann L. Whall*
*Dorothy Booth*

It has been estimated that 5% of the elderly population at any one time are residing in institutional settings (Butler & Lewis, 1982). The fact that the elderly population is continuing to grow indicates that the numbers that this 5% represents will be substantially increased in the future. We intend to concentrate in this chapter on nutrition and drug considerations for the elderly and the difference that an institutional setting makes. We define institutional setting for this discussion as including long-term moderate- to total-care facilities, regardless of organizational structure or financial support. We will use the terms *institutional setting* and *nursing care facility* interchangeably.

## NUTRITIONAL CONCERNS IN THE INSTITUTIONAL SETTING

Although most nursing care facilities (NCFs) attempt to provide a nutritionally sound diet, there are factors in the institutional setting itself and in those people who need institutional care that tend to conflict with adequate nutritional intake. Elderly persons who are in an institutional setting, for the most part, have chronic illnesses and are no longer able to manage their own care. In this group are also found a certain number who might be able to manage their care outside of the institution, were the needed support for staying in the community available to them.

Before institutionalization, the elderly residents were used to certain meal routines and certain foods of their own choosing. In addition, they were able to take prescription drugs as well as over-the-counter drugs in a routine that was tailored to their likes and dislikes. This may or may not have been a sound procedure in terms of the drugs involved. The newly admitted persons often were more physically active prior to admission than they are in the NCF. In addition, medications that had been prescribed when the elderly person was in the community may or may not have been managed effectively. Some of these medications may have interfered with the person's nutritional status, such as the use of mineral oil as a laxative. Many persons have had poor dietary habits all of their lives. For a few, poor dietary intake may have been related to lack of funds or an inability to procure food because of lack of transportation and/ or other factors such as high crimes rates. More than half of all persons over age 65 have no natural teeth, therefore, lack of dentures or ill fitting dentures may contribute to malnourishment. These factors, when taken together, often result in an individual being institutionalized who is malnourished and has established dietary preferences and accustomed drug routines.

Often the relocation is not an ideal choice, from the perspective of the elderly person, who may in fact be seeking care or be forced into an institution as a last resort. Once in the NCF, there is no longer as much freedom to come and go, to prepare meals in the usual manner, and to manage drug routines. A feeling of loss and a state of depression often appear soon after admission or are present at the time of admission. Depression is often related to loss of appetite. Add to this the fact that a drug regimen is often instituted to alleviate the person's depression, and we see a situation developing that may further compound the problems of a nutritionally unsound dietary intake and adverse drug–food interactions.

Many drugs that are useful in alleviating cardiac problems, hypertension, and a variety of other conditions can produce gastrointestinal symptoms that are related to a decrease in appetite. If the person is also given a low-salt or sugar-free diet, the food may not taste the same or be as palatable to the elderly person as the diet previously available. Further, the elderly person may have been used to eating in relative solitude, whereas in the NCF she or he probably will eat in a community situation which may be noisy and confusing. This change, along with the necessity of being close to new persons with a variety of physical and sometimes confusional conditions, often results in decreased appetite. From our perspective we see the problem of a sound nutritional intake for the elderly in an institutional setting to be less a problem of intent and more a problem of situation.

Some approaches to these problems are suggested by this conceptualization, from a need to do a complete dietary and drug assessment that takes into account individual preferences, to exercise programs that not only help alleviate depression but also may help improve appetite and decrease bowel problems. The esthetic factor, or mixing confused with nonconfused residents during meal times, is also a concern. More attention to this factor may decrease the adjustment needed to be made by nonconfused persons.

## CASE EXAMPLE

A hypothetical case example will serve as a transition between the beginning discussion of dietary factors in the care of the institutionalized elderly and discussion of the interaction effect of drugs and food in this setting. Although hypothetical, the material is drawn from several actual case examples.

Mrs. Smith was on drugs for a cardiac problem prior to admission to the NCF. The primary reason for her admission was a diagnosis of early Parkinson's disease and the lack of any close relative available to assist her at home. Upon admission, Mrs. Smith revealed her appetite was poor and she had lost approximately five pounds over the past year. She complained about a metallic taste in her mouth, which she related to her loss of appetite. When at home, however, she had been able to cover up the taste with various seasonings that were available to her when she cooked her own food. Closer inspection revealed that this metallic taste was a side effect of one of the cardiac drugs that she was taking. She was continued on the drug because it seemed the best one in terms of the cardiac condition.

Upon admission Mrs. Smith also was given an antiparkinsonian agent, which she noted tended to make her drowsy. At the appointed meal times Mrs. Smith was often noted to "doze" through meals without eating, though the staff attempted to wake her and assist her. Her caloric intake was further reduced, and she continued to lose weight. During this time her fluid intake also was reduced, perhaps because of her drowsiness, and she developed hard stools for the first time in her life. A stool softener was prescribed to manage the constipation, although she complained of a bitter taste in her mouth. Subsequently, she ate even less. Mrs. Smith, it was noted, was becoming more depressed, so an antidepressant drug was added to the drug regimen.

At this point, three months after admission, Mrs. Smith had lost a total of 12 pounds. She now was 5'5" tall and weighed 100 pounds. It was noted that she was intermittently confused throughout the day, asking to be shown to her kitchen; she also was intermittently incontinent of urine. One week later she was unable to feed herself; the following 2 weeks she was constantly confused. Mrs. Smith eventually lapsed into a coma and died 4 months after admission.

This is not an unusual vignette. One of the major features in this scenario, however, is the nutritional problems that were compounded by the medication routine. Medications sometimes are given at the same dosage as might have been given to a 200-pound middle-aged person. The dosage of the drugs, as well as Mrs. Smith's chronological age, may not have been taken into consideration. Since guidelines for administration of drugs to the elderly are sometimes not available, observing the patient closely for side effects and reducing dosages, changing drugs, or eliminating unnecessary drugs all become very important. Besides simplifying the drug routine, listening to Mrs. Smith's reasons for not eating, changing or eliminating drugs to overcome the problems, and letting her identify the seasonings she wanted would have gone a long way toward avoiding or changing the outcome of this scenario.

## DRUG CONCERNS IN THE INSTITUTIONAL SETTING

The most commonly used drugs for the elderly in institutions, both in terms of the literature and in our experience, are cathartics/stool softeners, analgesics, cardiovascular agents, hypertensives, hypnotics, and psychoactives. Simonson (1984) has noted many drug–food interactions can occur from the use of these types of medications. If mineral oil is used there will be a decreased absorption of oil-soluble vitamins. If monoamine oxidase inhibitors are used for depression, foods containing tyramine may cause a hypertensive crisis. In addition, the presence or absence of food in the stomach tends to alter the rate and amount of drug absorption into the bloodstream. This was an important consideration in Mrs. Smith's case.

"Blood thinners" are frequently prescribed for nursing home residents (e.g., warfarin). Simonson noted that the activity of warfarin is dependent on the presence or absence of Vitamin K. Excessive ingestion of foods higher in Vitamin K content (lean meat and green leafy vegetables) may lead to interactions with this drug. In addition, the elderly are often susceptible to peripheral vascular fragility, and large hematomas resulting from the use of blood thinners may result in care problems as well as concern on the part of the patient.

Because the elderly are often malnourished when they enter an institution, they may be particularly responsive to the effects of drugs. This is because the electrolytes and other laboratory values may be significantly different for the malnourished, and drug reactions may be very different from that of other populations. Lamy (1982) noted that drugs also may lead to subclinical malnutrition through the suppression of the appetite. Because gastric emptying and intestinal transit times result in altered uptake of drugs, Lamy noted that drug intoxication is more likely in the elderly. Such drugs as cardiac glycosides, administered chronically, can cause thiamine deficiency. Aspirin, it has been noted, may deplete a patient of folic acid. It also has been suggested that deficiencies of B vitamins can lead to pseudo-senility in older adults. In addition, a calcium/magnesium supplement often taken by women contains a number of toxic metals (Lamy, 1982).

To summarize, drug usage is increased in the elderly in an effort to overcome some of their chronic illnesses. This often occurs when they are malnourished and the drugs therefore have a more potent effect. Crooks (1983b) summarizes points that could help with nutrition/drug interactions that occur in institutional settings:

1. Is drug therapy needed?
   a. Many diseases from which the elderly suffer may be handled in a variety of ways.
   b. Do not, however, withhold drugs because of age, if appropriate drug treatment is needed.
   c. Use only needed drugs.
   d. Drug regimens should be reviewed regularly.
   e. Remember that drugs themselves may cause a variety of iatrogenic conditions, side effects, and synergistic effects.
2. Choose the appropriate drug.
   a. Drugs suitable for younger persons may have side effects in the elderly.
   b. Consider the form of drug (from syrup to size of pill).
3. Consider the dosage and regimen.
   a. In general give smaller doses.
   b. Once-a-day dosages are suggested because of less opportunity for error.
4. Give medication instructions.
   a. Patients should know the drug, the correct dose, and how to administer it. If they appear confused, repetition is necessary.

b. Drugs should be clearly labeled and in appropriate containers.
c. Supervision of therapy is important.

Polypharmacy in institutional settings has been identified in nursing research as a problem. Brown et al. (1977) studied drug interactions among residents in homes for the elderly; they found that of 188 residents in two homes, each resident received an average of six drugs. In the two institutions, 100 residents (or better than half of the number of residents in the two facilities) were identified as having potential drug-interaction problems. The drugs most often prescribed in these homes were, in rank order, (1) analgesics for arthritis, (2) laxatives for GI disturbances, (3) cardiovascular drugs, (4) psychotropics, and (5) vitamins. The most common potential drug interaction was between digitalis and the diuretics (a possible potassium-depletion situation). This potential interaction also was noted as a problem in two other studies. For preventive measures Brown et al. recommended a periodic evaluation of the drug effectiveness and of the continuing need for drugs. In their study they found that the use of tranquilizers, hypnotics, and sedatives was a potential hazard. Use of nondrug measures to quiet and relieve discomfort was recommended, as was an ongoing early detection system to identify potential drug interactions. It was suggested that drug profiles of each patient be available and reviewed regularly.

Hanan (1978) noted that many aging persons whose health and reserves are only marginal may be pushed over the brink by unneeded drug therapy into confusion, incompetence, and helplessness. He noted that all drugs ingested eventually pass through the liver. He added that the liver's capacity to metabolize decreases with age and that unmetabolized drugs continue to exert their effects. Drugs that are deactivated by the liver in younger patients (e.g., barbiturates and tricyclics) may cause prolonged effects in the elderly. He noted also that glomerular filtration rates are slowed in the elderly and that this, combined with a higher proportion of fat to total body weight, may result in even moderate dosages of drugs accumulating to toxic levels.

Comfort (1983) essentially agrees with this view when he states that there is no such thing in old age as a minor tranquilizer and there is no such thing as an acceptable long-term hypnotic for the elderly. In his opinion, of all the misused medications, the psychoactives probably rank first. Phenothiazines, he asserts, can produce as well as alleviate nocturnal confusion. Administered often in an understaffed nursing home, they may present as a good imitation of chronic brain syndrome. In addition, drugs are often prescribed and seldom are discontinued in the institutional setting.

Hicks, Funkenstein, Davis, and Dysken (1980) stated that generally the pharmacological effects of aging are prolongation of drug-elimination half-life, inconsistent changes in the volume of the distribution, increase in unbound drug, and decreased clearance of the drug from the kidneys. For these reasons more drug reactions are likely to occur with the aged. He identified levodopa absorption as being impaired when given with tricyclic antidepressants. This was a concern in the case of Mrs. Smith.

Periodic medication reviews have been used to monitor drug intake, watching especially "p.r.n." medications in institutional settings. A study by Howard, Strong, Strong, & Strong (1977) showed that, in the institutional setting, residents were receiving an average of 5.5 drugs. Fifty-eight percent of all these drugs were of the p.r.n. variety or dispensed at the discretion of the staff, who may or may not be well trained and knowledgeable. They found aspirin was the most commonly prescribed p.r.n. drug, followed by milk of magnesia. The review of prescriptions also revealed that laboratory tests for electrolytes were seldom ordered for patients receiving digitalis and diuretics. Hematocrit also was not ordered on a regular basis for patients who had recently suffered blood loss. They concluded that periodic review of medication orders by regulatory agencies was not sufficient, that an ongoing medication review similar to that suggested by Crooks (1983a) is needed. In this regard, Block (1982) suggested the use of computer assisted analysis to identify potential drug interactions, along with a high suspicion level on the part of staff.

In summary, individual and environmental interactions need to be considered when the elderly person enters an NCF. The smallest possible number of drugs should be used, and the dosage adjusted to fit the person's size, age, and weight. The staff needs to be aware of drug interactions and the response of elderly persons to certain classes of drugs. The elderly person should also be observed carefully and drug reviews done regularly to monitor for potential drug problems.

# 12
# Adherence to Treatment among the Elderly

## Jacqueline Dunbar

An examination of the use of drug and diet treatments among the elderly would be incomplete without consideration of their compliance to diet or drug prescriptions. Before we look at compliance specifically in this group, however, we need to put the problem of compliance in a broader perspective. While compliance with medical regimens has been the subject of intense study over the past decade, the study of compliance as a broader issue in human behavior actually began long before that.

In 1934, Allport published a paper describing the compliance or conforming behaviors of ordinary citizens to certain "rules of living." He considered such behaviors as stopping at stop lights, arriving at work on time, and the extent to which church rituals are carried out. Looking at the distribution of compliance rates, Allport made a very interesting discovery. He found that, for each of the behaviors examined, the majority of people complied most of the time: that is, stopped at traffic lights, arrived at work on time, and carried out church rituals. Others complied partially; that is, they slowed down before going through stop lights, were slightly late for work, and completed most of the rituals. The remainder never or rarely complied. When fre-quency-of-difference compliance rates were plotted, the resulting curve resembled the letter J. That is, most of the people complied most of the time, some complied partially, and still others rarely or never did. Based on this finding, Allport postulated the "J-curve hypothesis of conforming behavior."

Interestingly, the compliance rate for medical regimens seems to follow that same J-shaped distribution, with occasionally a shift toward the noncompliance end resulting in a U-shaped distribution. The J- or U-shaped compliance-rate distribution is found for a variety of regimens, including medication intake, diet interventions, and exercise prescriptions. Further, it is found in the treatment of both acute and chronic conditions, in simple medication interventions and more complex regimens, in preventive regimens and treatments for life-threatening conditions, and among adults caring for themselves and among parents caring for their children (Dunbar, 1980; Dunbar & Agras, 1980). Thus, the problem of noncompliance permeates medical care.

The elderly are no different. Indeed, the noncompliance rates among the elderly are similar to those for other age groups. More than 50% do not take drugs as prescribed (Ouslander, 1981). Approximately 5 to 15% are hospitalized as a result of medication errors (Gryfe & Gryfe, 1984). A recent study by Klein, German, McPhee, Smith, and Levine (1982) specifically examined the issue of age as a factor in patient adherence. The investigators identified patients over the course of nine months who were being discharged from the general medical service at Johns Hopkins Hospital and who were to be followed in the outpatient setting. Two hundred and sixty-five persons below the age of 65 and 139 persons 65 and over, who in combination were taking 970 long-term medications, were interviewed by telephone one month following discharge. Adherence data were collected by way of self-report, using a structured 15-minute multiple-choice interview. Data were collected on medication taken the day preceding the interview and were compared with what had been prescribed at discharge. As shown in Table 12.1, no significant difference between age groups in terms of compliance with medical instructions was found, even after controlling for the number of medications each person took.

A digression is appropriate here, regarding the assessment of adherence. Self-report, as used by Klein et al. (1982), is a com-

**TABLE 12.1**
**The Relationship of Age to Patient Compliance**

|  | % Compliant | |
| --- | --- | --- |
|  | <65 yrs. (n = 265) | ≥65 yrs. (n = 139) |
| Frequency of Medication Taking | 57.8% | 52.5% |
| Quantity of Medication Taken | 68.8% | 65.4% |

*Source*: Adapted from L. E. Klein, P. S. German, S. J. McPhee, C. R. Smith, and D. M. Levine. (1982). Aging and its relationship to health knowledge and medication compliance. *The Gerontologist, 22*(4), 384–397. Used by permission.

monly used method of eliciting adherence information. It does, however, tend to overestimate adherence, due to (1) the patient's unwillingness to report deviance, (2) the patient's faulty memory for the period covered by the assessment, and (3) difficulty in assessing one's own behavior. Klein et al. took steps to minimize these errors. For example, these investigators used only the day before the interview as the period of interest, thus minimizing potential memory problems that would arise with longer periods. The investigators further enhanced the accuracy of the self-report by using a structured interview rather than the more typical clinical assessment question, "Are you taking your medication or following your diet?"

While self-report may have its problems, two more common measures—clinical judgment and therapeutic response— should *not* be used as measures of adherence. Clinical judgment suffers serious validity problems; in fact, studies show that clinician judgments regarding patient adherence are no better than chance guesses, even when the clinician knows the patient well, is experienced, and/or is confident of his judgment (Roth, Caron, & Hsi, 1971). Therapeutic response is also not a reliable indicator of adherence, for a patient can comply without seeing clinical benefit (wrong prescription) or can fail to comply fully and yet see therapeutic benefit.

Given that the compliance rates in the elderly are similar to those of individuals in other age categories, one might ask whether the factors that contribute to nonadherence in the elderly are similar to those seen in other age groups. Indeed, this seems to be the case. One such factor is side effects. For example, the postural hypotension or impotence seen with certain of the antihypertensive drugs may lead individuals to stop medication. Lack of recall of the regimen is also a problem for all age groups. Further, the well-meaning advice from nonmedical persons, including family and relatives, may interfere with accurate adherence to the regimen. The communication skills and teaching ability of prescribing clinicians are important factors for all age groups. Cost factors also may preclude full compliance. Knowledge of the regimen is critical to compliance, yet studies show that many patients do not have the knowledge necessary to comply (Boyd, Covington, Stanaszck, & Coussins, 1974; Hulka, Cassell, & Kupper, 1976). In addition, the complexity of the regimen is critical. Transportation is a major factor in determining whether or not the individual can make office visits or clinic visits. The organization of the office or clinic delivering the services is a contributing factor, as are the amount of social support and the supervision offered for following the particular medication or dietary regimens. There is increasing evidence of the significance of a concept referred to as *self-efficacy*, that is, the personal belief that one can follow the regimen, as well as *therapeutic efficacy*, the belief that the treatment actually works. Both self-efficacy and therapeutic efficacy are important in determining regimen compliance (Schafer, Glasgow, McCaul, & Dreher, 1983). Related to this is how the individual weighs the cost-benefit ratio in deciding whether or not to comply. A hopeless, "what's the use" attitude may develop, particularly among the elderly, the depressed, or the chronically ill, related to lack of confidence in the treatment, excessive interference with what are perceived to be the few remaining pleasures of life, and even lack of desire to prolong one's own life. Each of these factors is important for any age group, including the elderly.

Three factors seem to be more specific to the elderly than to other age groups. First is the problem of mental status. Patients who are confused or who score poorly on mental status examinations do not do as well as other patients (MacDonald, MacDonald, & Pheonix, 1977). Fortunately, this includes a relative minority of the elderly. A second factor is that of decreased attention, which occurs with aging. Furthermore, the sensory declines that accompany aging may be related to compliance difficulties. For example, declines in visual acuity may lead to difficulties reading prescription labels or discriminating between different tablets. Declines in taste acuity may contribute to difficulties in adjusting to new dietary regimens.

A major factor, as noted, is the individual patient's comprehension of the regimen that has been prescribed. Three studies have examined the comprehension of elderly patients as it relates to regimen nonadherence. In these studies one fifth to one half of patients have difficulty understanding or lack knowledge about their medication regimen (Fletcher, Fletcher, Thomas, & Hamann, 1979; Parkin, Henney, Quirk, & Crooks, 1976; Schwartz et al., 1962). Some of the figures from these studies are presented in Table 12.2. The major problem was lack of knowledge of the particular dosage schedule, with only 58% of patients remembering this component of their regimen (Fletcher et al., 1979). Identifying the medication also appeared to be problematic: 19% of the patients were unable to identify the appropriate medication (Fletcher et al., 1979).

The question is, is this different from younger patients? Klein et al. (1982), as noted earlier, interviewed patients above and below age 65. They found a significant difference in knowledge of the purpose of specific medications between age groups: 54.5% of the older age group knew the purpose of the medications that had been prescribed, compared to 68.9% of the younger age group. This difference held even when differences in the number of prescribed medications had been taken into

**TABLE 12.2**
**Comprehension as a factor in Nonadherence in the Elderly**

| | |
|---|---|
| Fletcher et al. (1979) | 42% unaware of dosage schedule |
| | 35% unaware of purpose of medication |
| | 19% unable to identify medication |
| Parkin et al. (1976) | 35% did not understand regimen |
| Schwartz et al. (1962) | 20% of medication errors unaccounted for by inaccurate knowledge |

account. Interestingly, for both age groups knowledge of the purpose of the medication decreased as the number of drugs increased. In examining the older patients taking one drug versus those taking two to three drugs versus those taking four or more drugs, knowledge of the purpose of the medication was 75%, 52.3%, and 40.4%, respectively. The same trend was seen among the younger age group, although the knowledge level was higher, with the corresponding percentages being 86.9%, 59.9%, and 56.6%. It appears that the complexity of the regimen as defined by number of drugs taken and age are factors in comprehension of a medication regimen.

From the findings by Klein et al. (1982), it appears that patients ought to be educated about their regimens. Interestingly, the information that patients require is not information about the disease itself but information about the specific therapeutic regimen. No studies as yet have shown that information regarding the nature of the disease enhances compliance. The content of patient education thus needs to focus on the regimen itself.

In educating patients with the goal of improving their adherence to their therapeutic regimen, the amount of knowledge the patient retains can be enhanced by considering certain principles (Ley, Bradshaw, Eaves, & Walker, 1973). First, it is important to avoid overloading the patient. The more information transmitted to the patient, the less the patient remembers (Ley et al., 1973). That patients do forget information was shown in a classic study by Joyce, Capla, Mason, Reynolds, & Mathews (1969), in which patients were interviewed upon leaving the physician's office. He found that patients at that time had already lost two thirds of the information they had been given. A second factor in education is the importance of adapting teaching to the patient's level of attention. This is particularly true for the elderly patient, because the capacity for sustained attention declines with age. Third, the teaching needs to accommodate the sensory declines in the older patient. Acuity in eyesight and hearing declines as the patient ages; thus, small print and soft- or high-pitched voices tend to interfere with information acquired by the elderly. Fourth, memory aids can be utilized. As will be noted later, this needs to be handled with some caution.

Lastly, both the patient and any live-in caretaker or family member involved in the medication or dietary regimen of the patient need to understand the regimen.

Other than education, a number of additional adherence-enhancing techniques have been evaluated with the elderly. Among these are pharmacist counseling, the use of adherence aids, family involvement, alterations in drug packaging, and supervised practice before discharge.

Youngren (1981) did a study of the effect of supervised practice of medication intake before discharge, offering a self-medication teaching program to 32 hospitalized patients. The patients diagnosed as having chronic obstructive pulmonary disease were alert and cooperative and had no physical disabilities that could interfere with adherence. The teaching program included a description of the drug; its expected action, side effects, and dosage; and a medication schedule. The patients also were given a written handout containing the same information. Medication and the medication record were left at the patients' bedsides, first for administration under supervision and then for self-administration. Twenty-six of the 32 patients (81%) completed the program with 100% accuracy. Three patients had minor errors, and three could not self-administer the medication without assistance. Thus, the program had two potential benefits. First, patient medication errors could be corrected before the patient went home and was responsible for medication administration. Second, the program provided an opportunity to identify patients who would be unable to comply without assistance or supervision.

This type of program could be extended to dietary regimens as well. Activities such as shopping for special food items, menu planning, recipe adjustments, alterations in cooking, and so forth could be taught and subsequently performed under supervision before the patient was sent home to perform these tasks.

Drug packaging also has been examined as a factor in compliance among the elderly. Spriet, Beiler, Dechorgnat, & Simon (1980) analyzed 1,662 patients with cerebral symptoms such as impaired attention or memory loss, who were taking four tablets of pentoxifylline for a period of 4 weeks (Spriet et al., 1980). The patients were divided into four groups, and each group received one of four types of medication packages: (1) a box containing 40 tablets, (2) a box of 40 tablets plus red-label memory aids, (3) four tinfoil strips of 10 tablets each, and (4) four tinfoil strips of 10 tablets each plus red-label memory aids. Compliance was assessed by pill count (a measure that also is biased toward overreporting of good adherence). The compliance rates at the end of the four-week time period were as follows: 36.9% of the total sample were at 100% compliance, 25.3% ranged from 74 to 99% compliance; 12.4% ranged between 47 and 73%; and 8.5% were below 46% compliance. There were no differences in compliance rates among the types of packaging; however, the authors suspected that patients may not have returned partially filled or partially used containers. There tended to be peaks of medications returned at multiples of 10 for the tinfoil strips and 40 for the boxes. There were no effects noted for age, sex, number of medications prescribed, or other therapies.

The role of family involvement as an adherence enhancer was examined in a case report by Coe, Prendergast, & Psathas (1984). The results of this study supported the active involvement of family members in the direct administration or supervision of the regimen, if the patient was unable to take the medication himself or preferred to give up active involvement. Support for family involvement also can be derived from studies in dietary compliance. In the National Diet Heart Study (Archer, Rinzler, & Christakis, 1967) correlational data suggested that married men tended to comply with diet more than single men. Further, the weight-loss literature supports the active involvement of the spouse in the attainment and maintenance of weight loss (Pearce, LeBow, & Orchard, 1981). Further investigation would certainly be warranted in this particular area.

Other adherence aids have had mixed effects with the elderly. A variety of these aids have been evaluated in a number of studies. As noted earlier, Spriet et al. (1980) examined the use of special packaging, reminder stickers, and the use of special packaging enhanced with stickers. No effect for any of these packaging or reminder adherence aids was found. Martin and Mead (1982) also looked at packaging as an adherence aid. They found no improvement in compliance with the use of color-coded bottles, but they did find some improvement with the combined use of color-coded bottles plus color-coded pillboxes. MacDonald et al. (1977) examined the use of a pill-wheel container, a tablet identification card, and a tear-off daily reminder calendar. None of these had any noticeable effect on compliance. Wandless and Davie (1977), however, examined the use of a daily tear-off calendar and tablet identification cards and noted that both of these tended to improve compliance. A positive effect for daily drug-reminder charts also was noted by Gabriel, Gagnon, & Bryan (1977), who reported a 26% increase in mean compliance. Thus, the effect of adherence aids has not been consistent. The daily drug calendar seems to have the most support as a positive adherence aid.

When these aids are compared with simple adherence counseling alone, they do not do as well. For example, MacDonald et al. (1977) studied the effects of counseling plus medication aids with 165 consecutively discharged geriatric patients. These patients were divided into two groups, "oriented" and "confused," based upon a cutoff score of 12 on a mental-status questionnaire. Sixty patients, half of whom were oriented and half of whom were confused, served as controls; and 60 patients, half of whom were oriented and half of whom were confused, were studied in a counseling condition in which they received 15 minutes of counseling by the pharmacist at the time of discharge. The counseling included instruction on the name of the medication, the dose, and the time of administration. Forty-five patients served in a counseling-plus-adherence-aid condition. Counseling was identical to that received by the counseling-only group. In addition, these patients received a pinwheel medication container with a compartment for each day's medication, a tear-off calendar that noted each day's drug schedule, and tablet identification cards that included a picture of a pill and a schedule for that pill. Adherence was assessed for all three groups at 1 week and 12 weeks following discharge, and the data for each treatment group were isolated according to the mental-status score.

As can be seen from Figure 12.1, compliance deteriorated over time for all groups. The patients who were oriented did considerably better on compliance than those who were confused; however, both the oriented and confused patients im-

FIGURE 12.1 Effect of Medication Counseling on Oriented and Confused Patients, 1 Week and 12 Weeks after Discharge.

| | Percent of Patients Taking Medications Correctly | | | |
|---|---|---|---|---|
| | Mental Status Score≥12 | | Mental Status Score<12 | |
| Uncounseled | 46% | 34.6% | 23.5% | 14.7% |
| Counseled | 90.5% | 80% | 48.7% | 38.5% |
| Counseled + Aids | 75% | 60% | 68% | 24.0% |

◄━━ Adherence at 1 week

━━► Adherence at 12 weeks

*Source*: Adapted from E. T. MacDonald, J. B. MacDonald, and M. Phoenix (1977). Improving drug compliance after discharge. *British Medical Journal, 2,* 618–621, Tables I, II, and III. Data used with permission.

proved in their compliance through counseling or counseling plus adherence aids. Interestingly, of these two conditions, counseling alone appeared to be more effective than counseling plus aids. It should be noted that no data were presented on the extent of compliance with the counseling aids themselves, or whether patients found the aids confusing.

MacDonald et al. (1977) also examined comprehension as it related to compliance in this elderly population. Patients in the counseling-only and counseling-plus-aids conditions were given a comprehension assessment at the end of the counseling session. The relationship of initial comprehension of the medication schedule to adherence 12 weeks after the counseling session was then examined. Both the number of different types of errors as well as the total number of errors were considered. Errors were found to be of four types: underdosage, overdosage, use of outdated medication, and use of other people's medications. The average number of categories that contained errors was approximately the same with moderate and good comprehension, that is, .59 in the moderate group and .49 in the good group. Patients with poor comprehension were more likely to make multiple types of errors. This suggests that, in the education of patients regarding their drug regimens, lack of comprehension accounts for a certain amount of noncompliance. It is important to evaluate and insure the patient's comprehension at the end of an instructional session.

Compliance, of course, is not solely a function of patient errors. The problem needs to be seen in the context of a system of specialization in medical care where patients are likely to see more than one provider on a routine basis, each of whom may prescribe medication. In a study by Fletcher et al. (1979), it was found that physicians were unaware of 21% of the medications their patients were taking. Thus, compliance difficulties may arise from multiple providers instructing and prescribing for the patient.

## SUMMARY

The factors that contribute to compliance problems among the elderly are complex, and the strategies that have been evaluated to improve compliance are limited. What can be done, then, at the initiation of a drug or dietary regimen to minimize compliance problems? First, one needs to be aware of all prescriptions from all providers before planning care. Second, one needs to consider the complexity of the regimen and impact on the patient's lifestyle. The regimen should be the simplest possible and, if possible, tailored to the patient's lifestyle. It should take into consideration the patient's mental status, cost factors, extent of family support and supervision available, and the potential problems introduced by the normal declines in sensory functioning that accompany aging. For example, changes in visual acuity may make it difficult for the elderly patient to discriminate between medication of light hues or to match "arrows" on childproof pill bottles (Atkinson, Gibson, & Andrews, 1978). Third, one needs to provide adequate instruction on the regimen and utilize aids that will enhance memory of the correct regimen. If possible, practice of self-management of the regimen under supervision is advisable, as it may provide the opportunity to correct errors or misconceptions. Attention to these steps should minimize potential adherence errors, but the clinician should continue to provide adequate follow-up care and supervision to detect and modify adherence problems that may arise with time. Finally, as noted by MacDonald et al. (1977), adherence tends to decline with time; therefore, adherence to a medical regimen is a factor in treatment that will require ongoing attention.

# References

Abraham, S., Carroll, M. D., Dresser, C. M., & Johnson, C. L. (1977a).
Dietary intake in persons 1-74 years of age in the United States. *Advance data from Vital and Health Statistics of the National Center for Health Statistics, No. 6.* Rockville, MD: Health Resources Administration.

Abraham, S., Carroll, M. D., Dresser, C. M., & Johnson, C. L. (1977b).
*Health and nutrition examination survey.* DHEW Publication No. (HRA) 77-1647. Washington, DC: U.S. Government Printing Office.

Abramowicz, M. (1981). Adverse interactions of drugs. In M. Abramowicz (Ed.), *Medical letter on drugs and therapeutics, 23*(5), 17–28.

Alexander, D. D. (1950). *Arthritis and common sense.* Boston: Humphries.

Allen, L. H. (1982). Calcium bioavailability and absorption: A review. *American Journal of Clinical Nutrition, 35,* 783–808.

Allport, F. H. (1934). The J-curve hypothesis of conforming behavior. *Journal of Social Psychology, 5,* 141–183.

Altschule, M. D. (1978). *Nutritional factors in general medicine: Effects of stress and distorted diets.* Springfield, IL: Charles C Thomas.

Alvares, A. P., Anderson, K. E., Conney, A. H., & Kappas, A. (1976). Interactions between nutritional factors and drug biotransformations in man. *Proceedings of National Academy of Sciences, USA, 73,* 2501–2504.

Alvares, A. P., Kappas, A., Eiseman, J. L., Anderson, K. E., Pantuck, C. B., Pantuck, E. J., Hsiao, K. C., Garland, W. A., & Conney, A. H. (1979). Intraindividual variation in drug disposition. *Clinical Pharmacology and Therapeutics, 26,* 407–419.

American Medical Association. (1983). Calcium channel blocking agents. A report of the Council on Scientific Affairs, Division of Scientific Analysis and Technology. *Journal of the American Medical Association, 250,* 2522–2524.

Anderson, K. E., Conney, A. H., & Kappas, A. (1979). Nutrition and oxidative drug metabolism in man: Relative influence of dietary lipids, carbohydrate, and protein. *Clinical Pharmacology and Therapeutics, 26,* 493–501.

Anderson, K. E., Conney, A. H., & Kappas, A. (1982). Nutritional influences on chemical biotransformations in humans. *Nutrition Reviews, 40,* 161–171.

Anderson, K. E., & Kappas, A. (1982). Hormones and liver function. In L. Schiff & E. R. Schiff (Eds.), *Diseases of the liver* (5th ed., pp. 167–235). Philadelphia: Lippincott.

Anderson, K. E., Kappas, A., Conney, A. H., Bradlow, H. L., & Fishman, J. (1984). The influence of dietary protein and carbohydrate on the principal oxidative biotransformations of estradiol in normal subjects. *Journal of Clinical Endocrinology and Metabolism, 59,* 103–107.

Anderson, K. E., Schneider, J., Pantuck, E. J., Pantuck, C. B., Mudge, G. H., Welch, R. M., Conney, A. H., & Kappas, A. (1983). Acetaminophen metabolism in subjects fed charcoal-broiled beef. *Clinical Pharmacology and Therapeutics, 34,* 369–374.

Andres, R. (1971). Aging and diabetes. *Medical Clinics of North America, 55,* 835–846.

Andres, R. (1981). Aging, diabetes, and obesity: Standards of normality. *Mount Sinai Journal of Medicine, 48,* 489–495.

Andres, R. (1985). Mortality and obesity: The rationale for age-specific height-weight tables. In R. Andres, E. L. Bierman, & W. R. Hazzard (Eds.), *Principles of geriatric medicine* (pp. 311–318). New York: McGraw-Hill.

Annas, G. (1984). The case of Mary Hier: When substituted judgement becomes sleight of hand. *Hastings Center Report, 14*(4), 23–25.

Archer, M., Rinzler, S., & Christakis, G. (1967). Social factors affecting participation in a study of diet and coronary heart disease. *Journal of Health and Social Behavior, 8,* 22–31.

Armstrong, W. A., Driever, C. W., & Hays, R. L. (1980). Analysis of drug-drug interactions in a geriatric population. *American Journal of Hospital Pharmacy, 37,* 385–387.

Atchley, R. C. (1975). Dimensions of widowhood in later life. *Gerontologist, 15*(2), 176–178.

Atkinson, L., Gibson, I., & Andrews, J. (1978). An investigation into the ability of elderly patients continuing to take prescribed drugs after discharge from hospital and recommendations concerning improving the situation. *Gerontology, 24,* 225–234.

Avissar, S., Egozi, Y., & Sokolovsky, M. (1981). Aging process decreases the density of muscarinic receptors in rat adenohypophysis. *Febs Letters, 133,* 275–278.

Avorn, J., & Soumerai, S. B. (1983). Improving drug-therapy decisions through educational outreach. *New England Journal of Medicine, 308,* 1457–1463.

Bakke, O. M., Aanderud, S., Syversen, G., Bassoe, H., & Myking, O. (1978). Antipyrine metabolism in anorexia nervosa. *British Journal of Clinical Pharmacology, 5,* 341-343.

Balant, L. P. (1984). Pharmacokinetics in the 1980's. *Clinical Therapeutics, 6,* 112-124.

Barrows, C. H., & Kokkenen, G. C. (1984). Nutrition and aging: Human and animal laboratory studies. In J. M. Ordy, D. Harman, & R. Alfin-Slater (Eds.), *Nutrition in gerontology* (pp. 279-322). New York: Raven.

Barrows, C. H., & Roeder, L. M. (1977). Nutrition. In C. E. Finch & L. Hayflick (Eds.), *Handbook of the biology of aging* (pp. 561-581). New York: Van Nostrand Reinhold.

Bauman, J. H., & Kimelblatt, B. J. (1982). Cimetidine as an inhibitor of drug metabolism: Therapeutic implications and review of the literature. *Drug Intelligence and Clinical Pharmacy, 16,* 380-386.

Becker, M. H., Haefner, D. P., Kasl, S. V., Kirscht, J. P., Maiman, L. A., & Rosenstock, I. M. (1977). Selected psychosocial models and correlates of individual health-related behaviors. *Medical Care, 15*(Suppl. 5), 27-46.

Belloc, N. B. (1973). Relationship of health practices and mortality. *Preventive Medicine, 2,* 67-81.

Belloc, N. B., & Breslow, L. (1972). Relationship of physical health status and health practices. *Preventive Medicine, 1,* 409-421.

Belloc, N. B., Breslow, L., & Hochstim, J. R. (1971). Measurement of physical health in a general population survey. *American Journal of Epidemiology, 93,* 328-336.

Bellville, J. W., Forrest, W. H. Jr., Miller, E., & Brown, B. W. Jr. (1971). Influence of age on pain relief from analgesics. *Journal of the American Medical Association, 217,* 1835-1841.

Bender, A. D. (1974). Pharmacodynamic principles of drug therapy in the aged. *Journal of the American Geriatrics Society, 22,* 296-303.

Bennett, W. M., Muther, R. S., Parker, R. A., Feig, P., Morrison, G., Golper, T. A., & Singer, I. (1980). Drug therapy in renal failure: Dosing guidelines for adults. *Annals of Internal Medicine, 93,* 62-89, 286-325.

Berardo, F. (1968). Widowhood status in the U.S.: Perspectives on a neglected aspect of the family life cycle. *Family Coordinator, 17,* 191-203.

Berardo, F. (1970). Survivorship and social isolation: The case of the aged widower. *Family Coordinator, 19,* 11-15.

Berkley, G. E. (1978). *Cancer: How to prevent it and how to help your doctor fight it.* Englewood Cliffs, NJ: Prentice-Hall.

Blaschke, T. F., Cohen, S. N., Tatro, D. S., & Rubin, P. C. (1981). Drug-drug interactions and aging. In L. F. Jarvik, D. J. Greenblatt, & D. Harman (Eds.), *Clinical pharmacology and the aged patient* (pp. 11-26). New York: Raven Press.

Blazer, D. G., Federspiel, C. F., Ray, W. A., & Schaffner, W. (1983). The risk of anticholinergic toxicity in the elderly: A study of prescribing practices in two populations. *Journal of Gerontology, 38,* 31–35.

Block, L. (1982). Polymedicine: Known and unknown drug interactions. *Journal of the American Geriatrics Society, 30*(11), 595–598.

Boyd, J. R., Covington, T. R., Stanaszck, W. F., & Coussins, R. T. (1974). Drug defaulting, Part I: Determinants of compliance. *American Journal of Hospital Pharmacy, 31,* 362–367.

Brennan, M. F. (1979). Metabolic response to surgery in the cancer patient. *Cancer, 43*(5 Suppl.), 2053–2064.

Brody, E. M., Kleban, M. H., & Moles, E. (1983). What older people do about their day-to-day mental and physical health symptoms. *Journal of the American Geriatrics Society, 31*(8), 489–498.

Brody, S. J., & Magel, J. S. (1984). DRG: The second revolution in health care for the elderly. *Journal of the American Geriatrics Society, 32*(9), 676–679.

Brotman, H. (1978). The aging of America: A demographic profile. *National Journal, 10*(40), 1622–27.

Brown, M., Boosinger, J., Henderson, M., Rife, S., Rustia, J., Taylor, O., & Young, W. (1977). Drug-drug interactions among residents in homes for the elderly: A pilot study. *Nursing Research, 26,* 47–52.

Bruni, P. J. (1985). Chelation therapy: Opposition stymied by lack of definitive studies. *Patient Care, 19,* 20–21.

Burchinsky, S. G. (1984). Neurotransmitter receptors in the central nervous system and aging: Pharmacological aspect (review). *Experimental Gerontology, 19,* 227–239.

Butler, R. N., & Lewis, M. I. (1982). *Aging and mental health: Positive psychosocial and biomedical approaches.* St. Louis: C. V. Mosby.

Calderini, G., Bonetti, A. C., Aldinio, A., Savoini, G., DiPerri, B., Biggio, G., Toffano, G. (1981). Functional interaction between benzodiazepine and GABA recognition sites in aged rats. *Neurobiology of Aging, 2,* 309–313.

Caliendo, M. A. (1981). *Nutrition and preventive health care.* New York: Macmillan.

Campbell, A., & Baldessarini, R. J. (1981). Effects of maturation and aging on behavioral responses to haloperidol in the rat. *Psychopharmacology, 73,* 219–222.

Campbell, T. C., & Hayes, J. R. (1974). Role of nutrition in the drug-metabolizing enzyme system. *Pharmacological Reviews, 26,* 171–197.

Capron, A. M. (1984). Ironies and tensions in feeding the dying. *Hastings Center Report, 14*(5), 32–35.

Caranasos, G. J., Stewart, R. B., & Cluff, L. E. (1974). Drug-induced illness leading to hospitalization. *Journal of the American Medical Association, 228,* 713–717.

Cassileth, B. R., Lusk, E. J., Strouse, T. B., & Bodenheimer, B. J. (1984). Contemporary unorthodox treatments in cancer medicine. *Annals of Internal Medicine, 101,* 105–112.

Castleden, C. M., George, C. F., Marcer, D., & Hallett, C. (1977). Increased sensitivity to nitrazepam in old age. *British Medical Journal, 1,* 10–12.

Centenarians. (1984, September 16). *Parade Magazine,* p. 21.

Chandra, R. K. (1983). Numerical and functional deficiency in T helper cells in protein-energy malnutrition. *Clinical and Experimental Immunology, 51,* 126–132.

Chernoff, R. (1979). Nutrition and the cancer patient. *Journal of the Canadian Dietetic Association, 40*(2), 139–149.

Chernoff, R., & Lipschitz, D. A. (1986). Total parenteral nutrition: Considerations in the elderly. In J. L. Rombeau & M. D. Caldwell (Eds.), *Clinical nutrition. Vol. II: Total parenteral nutrition.* Philadelphia: W. B. Saunders.

Chernoff, R., Mitchell, C. O., & Lipschitz, D. A. (1984). Assessment of the nutritional status of the geriatric patient. *Geriatric Medicine Today, 3*(5), 129–141.

Ching, N., Grossi, C., Zurawinsky, H., Jham, G., Angers, J., Mills, C., & Nealon, T. F. (1979). Nutritional deficiencies and nutritional support therapy in geriatric cancer patients. *Journal of the American Geriatrics Society, 27,* 491–494.

Coe, R. M., Prendergast, C. G., & Psathas, G. (1984). Strategies for obtaining compliance with medications regimens. *Journal of the American Geriatrics Society, 32,* 589–594.

Colbert, C., & Bachtell, R. S. (1981). Radiographic absorptiometry. In S. H. Cohn, (Ed.), *Non-invasive measurements of bone mass and their clinical application* (pp. 51–84). Boca Raton, FL: CRC Press.

Collins, K. J., & Exton-Smith, A. N. (1983). Thermal homeostasis in old age. *Journal of the American Geriatrics Society, 31,* 519–524.

Comfort, A. (1983). Keynote address at symposium on drugs and the elderly, Toronto, May 4–5, 1981. *Journal of Chronic Diseases, 36*(1), 117–120.

Conney, A. H. (1967). Pharmacological implications of microsomal enzyme induction. *Pharmacological Reviews, 19,* 317–366.

Conney, A. H., Pantuck, E. J., Hsiao, K. C., Garland, W. A., Anderson, K. E., Alvares, A. P., & Kappas, A. (1976). Enhanced phenacetin metabolism in human subjects fed charcoal-broiled beef. *Clinical Pharmacology and Therapeutics, 20,* 633–642.

Conrad, K. A., & Bressler, R. (Eds.) (1982). *Drug therapy for the elderly.* St. Louis: C. V. Mosby.

Coon, M. J. (1978). Oxygen activation in the metabolism of lipids, drugs, and carcinogens. *Nutrition Reviews, 36,* 319–328.

Copeland, E. M. (1983). The patient with malignancy. In R. W. Winters &

H. L. Greene (Eds.), *Nutritional support of the seriously ill patient* (pp. 231-250). New York: Academic Press.

Crooks, J. (1983a). Aging and drug disposition: Pharmacodynamics. *Journal of Chronic Diseases, 36,* 85-90.

Crooks, J. (1983b). Rational therapeutics in the elderly. *Journal of Chronic Diseases, 36,* 59-65.

Crooks, J., & Stevenson, I. H. (1981). Drug response in the elderly: Sensitivity and pharmacokinetic considerations. *Age and Ageing, 10,* 73-80.

Cusack, B., Kelly, J. G., Lavan, J., Noel, J., & O'Malley, K. (1980). Pharmacokinetics of lignocaine in the elderly. *British Journal of Clinical Pharmacology, 9,* 293-294.

D'Arcy, P. F. (1982). Drug interaction. In P. F. D'Arcy & J. P. Griffin (Eds.), *Iatrogenic diseases* (pp. 21-40). New York: Oxford University Press.

D'Arcy, P. F., & McElnay, J. C. (1983). Adverse drug reactions and the elderly patient. *Adverse Drug Reactions and Acute Poisoning Reviews, 2,* 67-101.

Davies, D. F., & Shock, N. W. (1950). Age changes in glomerular filtration rate, effective renal plasma flow, and tubular excretory capacity in adult males. *Journal of Clinical Investigation, 29,* 496-507.

Davies, D. S., & Thorgeirsson, S. S. (1971). Individual differences in the plasma half-lives of lipid soluble drugs in man. *Acta Pharmacologica et Toxicologica, 29,* 181-190.

Donaldson, S. S., & Lenon, R. A. (1979). Alterations of nutritional status: Impact of chemotherapy and radiation therapy. *Cancer, 43*(5 Suppl.), 2036-2052.

Draper, H. H., & Scythes, C. A. (1981). Calcium, phosphorous, and osteoporosis. *Federation Proceedings, 40,* 2434-2438.

Dunbar, J. (1980). Adherence to medical regimen: A review. *International Journal of Mental Health, 9,* 70-87.

Dunbar, J., & Agras, W. S. (1980). Compliance with medical regimen. In J. Ferguson & C. B. Taylor (Eds.), *Comprehensive handbook of behavioral medicine.* Jamaica, NY: Spectrum.

Eastman, P. (1984, December). The surprising appeal of quack medicine. *Medica,* pp. 24-27.

Edelman, N. H., Mittman, C., Norris, A. H., Cohen, B. H., & Shock, N. W. (1966). The effects of cigarette smoking upon spirometric performance on community dwelling men. *American Review of Respiratory Disease, 94,* 421-429.

Eraker, S. A., Kirscht, J. P., & Becker, M. H. (1984). Understanding and improving patient compliance. *Annals of Internal Medicine, 100*(2), 258-268.

Erikson, E. H. (1968). *Identity, youth and crisis.* New York: W. W. Norton.

Esko, E. (1981). *The cancer prevention diet: How to live longer, healthier and happier through macrobiotics.* Brookline, MA: East West Foundation.

Estabrook, R. W., Martinez-Zedillo, G., Young, S., Peterson, J. A., & McCarthy, J. (1975). The interaction of steroids with liver microsomal cytochrome p-450: A general hypothesis. *Journal of Steroid Biochemistry, 6,* 419–425.

Farrell, G. C., Cooksley, W. G. E., Hart, P., & Powell, L. W. (1978). Drug metabolism in liver disease. Identification of patients with impaired hepatic drug metabolism. *Gastroenterology, 75,* 580–588.

Fedder, D. O. (1982). Managing medication and compliance: Physician-pharmacist-patient interactions. *Journal of the American Geriatrics Society, 30*(Suppl. 11), S113–S117.

Feely, J., Pereira, L., Guy, E., & Hockings, N. (1984). Factors affecting the response to inhibition of drug metabolism by cimetidine: Dose response and sensitivity of elderly and induced subjects. *British Journal of Clinical Pharmacology, 17,* 77–81.

Feldman, C. H., Hutchinson, V. E., Pippenger, C. E., Blumenfeld, T. A., Feldman, B. R., & Davis, W. J. (1980). Effect of dietary protein and carbohydrate on theophylline metabolism in children. *Pediatrics, 66,* 956–962.

Feldman, R. D., Limbird, L. E., Nadeau, J., Robertson, D., & Wood, A. J. J. (1984). Alterations in leukocyte beta-receptor affinity with aging. *New England Journal of Medicine, 310,* 815–819.

Fisher, M., Weiner, B., Ockene, I. S., Levine, P. H., Hoogasian, J., Arsenault, J. R., Natale, A. M., Johnson, M. H., & Vandreiul, C. H. (1985). The effect of cod liver oil on platelets and prostaglandins. *Neurology, 35* (Suppl. 1), 142.

Fitzgerald, D., Doyle, V., Kelly, J. G., & O'Malley, K. (1984). Cardiac sensitivity to isoprenaline, lymphocyte beta-adrenoceptors and age. *Clinical Science, 66,* 697–699.

Fletcher, S. W., Fletcher, R. H., Thomas, D. C., & Hamann, C. (1979). Patients' understanding of prescribed drugs. *Journal of Community Health, 4*(3), 183–189.

Flombaum, C., Isaacs, M., Scheiner, E., & Vanamee, P. (1981). Management of fluid retention in patients with advanced cancer. *Journal of the American Medical Association, 245,* 611–614.

Fong, N. L. (1979). Chemotherapy and nutritional management. In J. J. Wollard (Ed.), *Nutritional management of the cancer patient* (pp. 69–82). New York: Raven Press.

Frazer, J. G. (1951). *The golden bough: A study in magic and religion.* New York: Macmillan.

Fries, J. F. (1984). The compression of morbidity: Miscellaneous comments about a theme. *The Gerontologist, 24,* 354–359.

Gabriel, M., Gagnon, J. P., & Bryan, C. K. (1977). Improved patient compliance through use of a daily drug reminder chart. *American Journal of Public Health, 67*(10), 968–969.

Gallagher, J. C., Riggs, B. L., Eisman, J., Hamstra, A., Arnaud, S. B., & DeLuca, H. F. (1979). Intestinal calcium absorption and serum vitamin D metabolites in normal subjects and osteoporotic patients: Effect of age and dietary calcium. *Journal of Clinical Investigation, 64,* 729–736.

Gambrell, R. D. Jr. (1982). The menopause: Benefits and risks of estrogen-progesterone replacement therapy. *Fertility and Sterility, 37,* 457–474.

Gardner, P., & Cluff, L. E. (1970). The epidemiology of adverse drug reactions: A review and perspective. *Johns Hopkins Medical Journal, 126,* 77–87.

Gershon, D. (1979). Current status of age altered enzymes: Alternative mechanisms. *Mechanisms of Ageing and Development, 9,* 189–196.

Giannetti, V. J. (1983). Medication utilization problems among the elderly. *Health and Social Work, 8,* 262–270.

Goldberg, P. B., & Roberts, J. (1983). Pharmacologic basis for developing rational drug regimens for elderly patients. *Medical Clinics of North America, 67,* 315–331.

Goldsmith, R. S., & Ingbar, S. H. (1966). Inorganic phosphate treatment of hypercalcemia of diverse etiologies. *New England Journal of Medicine, 274,* 1–7.

Gomolin, I. H., & Chapron, D. J. (1983). Rational drug therapy for the aged. *Comprehensive Therapy, 9*(7), 17–30.

Graham, S., & Mettlin, C. (1979). Diet and colon cancer. *American Journal of Epidemiology, 109,* 1–20.

Greenblatt, D. J., Abernethy, D. P., Morse, D. S., Harmatz, J. S., & Shader, R. I. (1984). Clinical importance of the interaction of diazepam and cimetidine. *New England Journal of Medicine, 310,* 1639–1643.

Greenblatt, D. J., Allen, M. D., & Shader, R. I. (1977). Toxicity of high dose flurazepam in the elderly. *Clinical Pharmacology and Therapeutics, 21,* 355–361.

Greenblatt, D. J., Sellers, E. M., & Shader, R. I. (1982). Drug disposition in old age. *The New England Journal of Medicine, 306,* 1081–1088.

Greene, H. L. (1983). A pathophysiologic approach to dietary management in patients with protracted diarrhea and malnutrition. In R. W. Winters & H. L. Greene (Eds.), *Nutritional support of the seriously ill patient* (pp. 181–194). New York: Academic Press.

Gregory, G. A., Eger, E. I., & Munson, E. S. (1969). The relationship between age and halothane requirement in man. *Anaesthesiology, 30,* 488–491.

Gryfe, C. I., & Gryfe, B. (1984). Drug therapy of the aged: The problem of compliance and the rules of physicians and pharmacists. *Journal of the American Geriatrics Society, 32*(4), 301–307.

Hammarlund, E. R., Ostrom, J. R., & Kethley, A. J. (1985). The effects of drug counseling and other educational strategies on drug utilization of the elderly. *Medical Care, 23*(2), 165-170.

Hanan, Z. (1978). Geriatric medications: How the aged are hurt by drugs meant to help. *R.N., 41,* 57-61.

Hathcock, J. N., & Coon, J. (1978). *Nutrition and drug interrelations.* New York: Academic Press.

Hayflick, L. (1980). Recent advances in the cell biology of aging. *Mechanisms of Ageing and Development, 14,* 59-79.

Hayflick, L. (1984). Intracellular determinants of cell aging. *Mechanisms of Ageing and Development, 28,* 177-185.

Haynes, R. B., & Sackett, D. L. (1976). *Compliance with therapeutic regimens.* Baltimore and London: Johns Hopkins University Press.

Haynes, R. B., Taylor, D. W., & Sackett, D. L. (Eds.). (1979). *Compliance in health care.* Baltimore: Johns Hopkins University Press.

Hazzard, W. R. (1984). Drug therapy of hyperlipidemia and obesity in the elderly: When the therapeutic ratio dips to unity. In R. E. Vestal, (Ed.), *Drug treatment in the elderly* (pp. 262-276). Sydney, Australia: ADIS Health Sciences Press.

Heaney, R. P., Gallagher, J. C., Johnston, C. C., Neer, R., Parfitt, A. M., & Whedon, G. D. (1982). Calcium nutrition and bone health in the elderly. *American Journal of Clinical Nutrition, 36,* 986-1013.

Heaney, R. P., Recker, R. R., & Saville, P. D. (1977). Calcium balance and calcium requirements in middle-aged women. *American Journal of Clinical Nutrition, 30,* 1603-1611.

Hicks, R., Funkenstein, H. H., Davis, J. M., & Dysken, M. W. (1980). Geriatric psychopharmacology. In J. E. Birren & R. B. Sloane (Eds.), *Handbook of mental health and aging* (pp. 745-774). Englewood Cliffs, NJ: Prentice-Hall.

Hitt, C. (1982, Jan-Feb). Risk reduction: A community strategy. *Community Nutritionist,* pp. 12-17.

Holland, J. C. B., Rowland, J., & Plumb, M. (1977). Psychological aspects of anorexia in cancer patients. *Cancer Research, 37,* 2425-2428.

Hollenberg, N. K., Adams, D. F., Solomon, H. S., Rashid, A., Abrams, H. L., & Merrill, J. P. (1974). Senescence and renal vasculature in normal man. *Circulation Research, 34,* 309-316.

Holliday, R., Huschtscha, L. I., Tarrant, G. M., & Kirkwood, T. B. L. (1977). Testing the commitment theory of cellular aging. *Science, 198,* 366-372.

Hollonbeck, D., & Ohls, J. C. (1984). Participation among the elderly in the food stamp program. *The Gerontologist, 24*(6), 616-621.

Howard, J., Strong, K. Sr., Strong, F., & Strong, K. Jr. (1977). Medication procedures in a nursing home: Abuse of PRN orders. *Journal of the American Geriatrics Society, 25*(2), 83-84.

Hulka, B. S., Cassell, J. C., & Kupper, L. L. (1976). Disparities between medications prescribed and consumed among chronic disease patients. In L. Lasagna (Ed.), *Patient compliance* (pp. 123–152). Mount Kisco, NY: Futura Publishing.

Hurwitz, N. (1969). Predisposing factors in adverse reactions to drugs. *British Medical Journal, I,* 536–539.

Ito, H. (1979). Age-related changes in insulin action and binding of $I^{125}$-insulin to the cultured human skin fibroblasts. *Journal of the Japanese Diabetic Society, 22,* 517–526.

James, O. F. W., Rawlins, M. D., & Woodhouse, K. (1982). Lack of aging effect on human microsomal monoxygenase enzyme activities and on inactivation pathways for reactive metabolic intermediates. In K. Kitani (Ed.), *Liver and aging* (pp. 395–406). Amsterdam: Elsevier.

Jarvik, L. F., Greenblatt, D. J., & Harman, D. (Eds.). (1981). *Clinical pharmacology and the aged patient.* New York: Raven Press.

Jarvik, L. F., & Kakkar, P. R. (1981). Aging and response to antidepressants. In L. F. Jarvik, D. J. Greenblatt, & D. Harman (Eds.), *Clinical pharmacology and the aged patient* (pp. 49–77). New York: Raven Press.

Jarvis, D. C. (1958). *Folk medicine: A Vermont doctor's guide to good health.* New York: Holt.

Jarvis, W. T. (1983). Food faddism, cultism, and quackery. *Annual Review of Nutrition, 3,* 35–52.

Jenne, J. Nagasawa, H., McHugh, R., MacDonald, F., & Wyse, E. (1975). Decreased theophylline half-life in cigarette smokers. *Life Sciences, 17,* 195–198.

Jick, H. (1974). Drugs: Remarkably nontoxic. *New England Journal of Medicine, 291,* 824–828.

Jovanovic, L., & Peterson, C. M. (Eds.). (1985). *Nutrition and diabetes.* New York: Alan R. Liss.

Joyce, C. R. B., Capla, G., Mason, M., Reynolds, E., & Mathews, J. A. (1969). Quantitative study of doctor-patient communication. *Quarterly Journal of Medicine, 38,* 183–194.

Judd, H. L., Cleary, R. E., Creasman, W. T., Figge, D. C., Kase, N., Rosenwaks, Z., & Tagatz, G. E. (1981). Estrogen replacement therapy. *Obstetrics and Gynecology, 58,* 267–275.

Judge, T. G., & Caird, F. I. (1978). *Drug treatment of the elderly patient.* Kent, England: Pitman Medical.

Kaiko, R. F. (1980). Age and morphine analgesia in cancer patients with postoperative pain. *Clinical Pharmacology and Therapeutics, 28,* 823–826.

Kalchthaler, T., Coccaro, E., & Lichtiger, S. (1977). Incidence of polypharmacy in a long-term care facility. *Journal of the American Geriatrics Society, 25,* 308–313.

Kalimi, M., & Seifler, S. (1979). Glucocorticoid receptors in W1-38 fibroblasts, characterization and changes with population doubling in culture. *Biochimica et Biophysica Acta, 583,* 352-359.

Kane, R. L., Ouslander, J. G., & Abrass, I. B. (1984). *Essentials of clinical geriatrics.* New York: McGraw-Hill.

Kappas, A., Alvares, A. P., Anderson, K. E., Pantuck, E. J., Pantuck, C. B., Chang, R., & Conney, A. H. (1978). Effect of charcoal-broiled beef on antipyrine and theophylline metabolism. *Clinical Pharmacology and Therapeutics, 23,* 445-450.

Kappas, A., Anderson, K. E., Conney, A. H., & Alvares, A. P. (1976). Influence of dietary protein and carbohydrate on antipyrine and theophylline metabolism in man. *Clinical Pharmacology and Therapeutics, 20,* 643-653.

Kappas, A., Anderson, K. E., Conney, A. H., Pantuck, E. J., Fishman, J., & Bradlow, H. L. (1983). Nutrition-endocrine interactions: Induction of reciprocal changes in the delta[4]-5-alpha-reduction of testosterone and the cytochrome p-450-dependent oxidation of estradiol by dietary macronutrients in man. *Proceedings of the National Academy of Sciences, USA, 80,* 7646-7649.

Kappas, A., Bradlow, H. L., Bickers, D. R., & Alvares, A. P. (1977). Induction of a deficiency of steroid delta[4]-5-alpha-reductase activity in liver by a porphyrinogenic drug. *Journal of Clinical Investigation, 59,* 159-164.

Kart, C. S. (1981). In the matter of Earle Spring: Some thoughts on one court's approach to senility. *The Gerontologist, 21*(4), 417-423.

Kart, C. S., & Metress, S. P. (1984). *Nutrition, the aged, and society.* Englewood Cliffs, NJ: Prentice-Hall.

Kato, R. (1978). Hepatic microsomal drug metabolizing enzymes in aged rats: History and future problems. In K. Kitani (Ed.), *Liver and aging* (pp. 287-299). Amsterdam: Elsevier.

Kelly, J. G., & O'Malley, K. (1979). Clinical pharmocokinetics of oral anticoagulants. *Clinical Pharmacokinetics, 4,* 1-15.

Kelly, J. G., & O'Malley, K. (1984). Adrenoceptor function and ageing. *Clinical Science, 66,* 509-515.

Kerr, I. G., & Chabner, B. A. (1983). The effect of age on the clinical pharmacology of anticancer drugs. In R. Yancik, P. P. Carbone, W. B. Patterson, K. Steel, & W. D. Terry (Eds.), *Perspectives on prevention and treatment of cancer in the elderly* (pp. 203-213). New York: Raven Press.

Keys, A., Brozek, J., Henschel, A., Mickelsen, O., & Taylor, H. L. (1950). The capacity for work. In A. Keys (Ed.), *The biology of human starvation* (Vol. 1, pp. 714-748). Minneapolis: University of Minnesota Press.

Kitani, K., Masuda, Y., Sato, Y., Kanai, S., Ohta, M., & Nokubo, M. (1984). Increased anticonvulsant effect of phenytoin in aging BDFI mice. *The Journal of Pharmacology and Experimental Therapeutics, 229,* 231-236.

Klein, L. E., German, P. S., McPhee, S. J., Smith, C. R., & Levine, D. M. (1982). Aging and its relationship to health knowledge and medication compliance. *The Gerontologist, 22*(4), 384–387.

Klotz, U., Avant, G. R., Hoyumpa, A., Schenker, S., & Wilkinson, G. R. (1975). The effects of age and liver disease on the disposition and elimination of diazepam in adult man. *Journal of Clinical Investigation, 55,* 347–359.

Kramer, P., & McClain, C. J. (1981). Depression of aminopyrine metabolism by influenza vaccination. *New England Journal of Medicine, 305*(21), 1262–1264.

Lamy, P. P. (1980). *Prescribing for the elderly.* Littleton, MA: PSC Publishing.

Lamy, P. P. (1982). Effects of diet and nutrition on drug therapy. *Journal of the American Geriatrics Society, 30*(11), S99–S112.

Lamy, P. P. (1983). Drug abuse by older adults: Who is responsible? *Drug Intelligence and Clinical Pharmacy, 17*(9), 657–659.

Lasagna, L. (1956). Drug effects as modified by aging. *Journal of Chronic Diseases, 3,* 567–574.

Ley, P., Bradshaw, P. W., Eaves, D., & Walker, C. M. (1973). A method for increasing patients' recall of information presented by doctors. *Psychological Medicine, 3,* 217–220.

Lindeman, R. (1982). Mineral metabolism in the aging and the aged. *Journal of the American College of Nutrition, 1,* 49–73.

Lindeman, R. D., Tobin, J., & Shock, N. W. (1984, June). *Longitudinal studies on the rate of decline in renal function with age.* Paper presented at the meeting of the Ninth International Congress of Nephrology, Los Angeles, CA.

Lindgren, S., Collste, P., Nordlander, B., & Sjögvist, F. (1974). Gas chromatographic assessment of the reproducibility of phenazone plasma half-life in young healthy volunteers. *European Journal of Clinical Pharmacology, 7,* 381–385.

Linkswiler, H. M., Joyce, C. L., & Anand, C. R. (1974). Calcium retention of young adult males as affected by level of protein and of calcium intake. *Transaction of the New York Academy of Sciences, 36,* 333–340.

Lippa, A. S., Critchett, D. J., Ehlert, F., Yamamura, H. I., Enna, S. J., & Bartus, R. T. (1981). Age-related alterations in neurotransmitter receptors: An electrophysiological and biochemical analysis. *Neurobiology of Aging, 2*(1), 3–8.

Lipschitz, D. A., Mitchell, C. O., & Thompson, C. (1981). The anemia of senescence. *American Journal of Hematology, 11,* 47–54.

Lotz, M., Zisman, E., & Bartter, F. C. (1968). Evidence for a phosphorus-depletion syndrome in man. *New England Journal of Medicine, 278,* 409–415.

Loub, W. D., Wattenberg, L. W., & Davis, D. W. (1975). Aryl hydrocarbon hydroxylases induction in rat tissues by naturally occurring indoles of cruciferous plants. *Journal of the National Cancer Institute, 54,* 985–988.

Lowenberg, M. E., Todhunter, E. N., Wilson, E. D., Feeney, M. C., & Savage, J. R. (1968). *Food and man.* New York: John Wiley.

Lundin, D. V. (1978). Medication taking behavior in the elderly: A pilot study. *Drug Intelligence and Clinical Pharmacy, 12,* 518–522.

MacDonald, E. T., MacDonald, J. B., & Phoenix, M. (1977). Improving drug compliance after hospital discharge. *British Medical Journal, 2,* 618–621.

Makinodan, T., James, S. J., Inamizu, T., & Chang, M. P. (1984). Immunologic basis for susceptibility to infection in the aged. *Gerontology, 30,* 279–289.

Margen, S., Chu, J. Y., Kaufmann, N. A., & Calloway, D. H. (1974). Studies in calcium metabolism, Part 1: The calciuretic effect of dietary protein. *American Journal of Clinical Nutrition, 27,* 584–589.

Martin, D. C., & Mead, K. (1982). Reducing medication errors in a geriatric population. *Journal of the American Geriatrics Society, 30*(4), 258–260.

Masoro, E. J. (1976). Physiologic changes with aging. In M. Winick (Ed.), *Nutrition and aging* (pp. 61–76). New York: John Wiley.

May, F. E., Stewart, R. B., Hale, W. E., & Marks, R. G. (1982). Prescribed and nonprescribed drug use in an ambulatory elderly population. *Southern Medical Journal, 75,* 522–528.

Mazess, R. B. (1982). On aging bone loss. *Clinical Orthopaedics and Related Research, 165,* 239–252.

McCarron, D. A., Morris, C. D., & Cole, C. (1982). Dietary calcium in human hypertension. *Science, 217,* 267–269.

McCarron, D. A., Morris, C. D., Henry, H. J., & Stanton, J. L. (1984). Blood pressure and nutrient intake in the United States. *Science, 224,* 1392–1398.

McGarry, K., Laher, M., Fitzgerald, D., Horgan, J., O'Brien, E., & O'Malley, K. (1983). Baroreflex function in elderly hypertensives. *Hypertension, 5,* 763–766.

McWhirter, N. D. (1983). *The Guinness book of world records.* New York: Bantam Books.

Mechnikov, I. I. (1908). *Prolongation of life: Optimistic studies.* New York: G. P. Putnam's Sons.

Meguid, M. M., Gray, G. E., & Debonis, D. (1984). The use of enteral nutrition in the patient with cancer. In J. L. Rombeau & M. D. Caldwell (Eds.), *Clinical nutrition, Vol. I: Enteral and tube feeding* (pp. 303–337). Philadelphia: W. B. Saunders.

Meilaender, G. (1984). On removing food and water: Against the stream. *Hastings Center Report, 14*(6), 11–13.

Metal chelation therapy, oxygen radicals, and human disease (editorial). (1985). *Lancet, 1,* 143–145.

Metropolitan Life Insurance Company. (1959). New weight standards for men and women. *Statistical Bulletin, 40*(11), 1–4.

Metropolitan Life Insurance Company. (1983). 1983 Metropolitan height and weight tables. *Statistical Bulletin, 64,* 2–9.

Mettlin, C., Graham, S., & Swanson, M. (1979). Vitamin A and lung cancer. *Journal of the National Cancer Institute, 62,* 1435–1438.

Miller, C. A., Slusher, L. B., & Vesell, E. S. (1985). Polymorphism of theophylline metabolism in man. *Journal of Clinical Investigation, 75,* 1415–1425.

Mitchell, C. O., & Lipschitz, D. A. (1982). Detection of protein-calorie malnutrition in the elderly. *American Journal of Clinical Nutrition, 35,* 398–406.

Mucklow, J. C., Caraher, M. T., Idle, J. R., Rawlins, M. D., Sloan, T., Smith, R. L., & Wood, P. (1980). The influence of changes in dietary fat on the clearance of antipyrine and 4-hydroxylation of debrisoquine. *British Journal of Clinical Pharmacology, 9,* 283P.

Munnell, A. H. (1977). *The future of social security.* Washington, DC: The Brookings Institution.

Myers, M. G., Weingert, M. E., Fisher, R. H., Gryfe, C. I., & Shulman, H. S. (1982). Unnecessary diuretic therapy in the elderly. *Age and Ageing, 11,* 213–221.

National Institutes of Health. (1979). *Diet and nutrition: A resource for parents of children with cancer.* NIH Publication No. 80-2038. Washington, DC: U.S. Government Printing Office.

National Institutes of Health. (1980). *Eating hints, recipes and tips for better nutrition during treatment.* NIH Publication No. 80-2079. Washington, DC: U.S. Government Printing Office.

National Research Council, Food and Nutrition Board. (1964). *Recommended dietary allowances, sixth edition.* Washington, DC: National Academy of Sciences.

National Research Council, Food and Nutrition Board. (1968). *Recommended dietary allowances* (7th ed.). Washington, DC: National Academy of Sciences.

National Research Council, Food and Nutrition Board. (1974). *Recommended dietary allowances* (8th rev. ed.). Washington, DC: National Academy of Sciences.

National Research Council, Food and Nutrition Board. (1980a). *Recommended dietary allowances* (9th rev. ed.). Washington, DC: National Academy of Sciences.

National Research Council, Food and Nutrition Board. (1980b). *Towards healthful diets.* Washington, DC: National Academy of Sciences.

Navia, J. M., & Harris, S. S. (1980). Vitamin A influence on calcium metabolism and calcification. In O. A. Levander, & L. Cheng (Eds.), *Micronutrient interactions: Vitamins, minerals, and hazardous elements* (Vol. 355 in the Annals of New York Academy of Sciences, pp. 45–57). New York: New York Academy of Sciences.

Nelson, G. (1982). Social class and public policy for the elderly. *Social Service Review, 56,* 85–107.

Newbold, H. L. (1979). *Vitamin C against cancer.* New York: Stein and Day.

Newmark, S. R., & Williamson, B. (1983). Survey of very-low-calorie weight reduction diets: Novelty diets. *Archives of Internal Medicine, 143,* 1195–1198.

O'Hanlon, P., & Kohrs, M. B. (1978). Dietary studies of older Americans. *American Journal of Clinical Nutrition, 31,* 1257–1269.

Ohlson, M. A., Jackson, J., Boek, J., Cederquist, D. C., Brewer, W. D., Brown, E. G., Traver, J., Lott, M. M., Mayhew, M., Dunsing, D., & Tobey, H. (1950). Nutrition and dietary habits of aging women. *American Journal of Public Health, 40,* 1101–1108.

Ohnuma, T., & Holland, J. F. (1977). Nutritional consequences of cancer chemotherapy and immunotherapy. *Cancer Research, 37,* 2395–2406.

Okada, A. A., & Dice, J. F. (1984). Altered degradation of intracellular proteins in aging human fibroblasts. *Mechanisms of Ageing and Development, 26,* 341–356.

O'Malley, K., Crooks, J., Duke, E., & Stevenson, I. H. (1971). Effect of age and sex on human drug metabolism. *British Medical Journal, 3,* 607–609.

O'Malley, K., Stevenson, I. H., Ward, C. A., Wood, A. J. J., & Crooks, J. (1977). Determinants of anticoagulant control in patients receiving warfarin. *British Journal of Clinical Pharmacology, 4,* 309–314.

Orme, M. L'E., & Tallis, R. C. (1984). Metoclopramide and tardive dyskinesia in the elderly. *British Medical Journal, 289,* 397–398.

Orshansky, M. (1978). *Testimony before U.S. House Select Committee on Aging: Poverty among America's aged.* Washington, DC: U.S. Government Printing Office.

Otten, A. L. (1984, July 30). The oldest old: Ever more Americans live into the 80s and 90s, causing big problems. *The Wall Street Journal,* p. 1.

Ouslander, J. G. (1981). Drug therapy in the elderly. *Annals of Internal Medicine, 95,* 711–722.

Oyeyinka, G. O. (1984). Age and sex differences in immunocompetence. *Gerontology, 30,* 188–195.

Pantuck, E. J., Hsiao, K. C., Kuntzman, R., & Conney, A. H. (1975). Intestinal metabolism of phenacetin in the rat: Effect of charcoal-broiled beef and rat chow. *Science, 187,* 744–746.

Pantuck, E. J., Hsiao, K. S., Maggio, A., Nakamura, K., Kuntzman, R., & Conney, A. H. (1974). Effect of cigarette smoking on phenacetin metabolism. *Clinical Pharmacology and Therapeutics, 15*, 9–17.

Pantuck, E. J., Pantuck, C. B., Anderson, K. E., Wattenberg, L. W., Conney, A. H., & Kappas, A. (1984). Effect of brussels sprouts and cabbage on drug conjugation. *Clinical Pharmacology and Therapeutics, 35*, 161–169.

Pantuck, E. J., Pantuck, C. B., Garland, W. A., Min, B. H., Wattenberg, L. W., Anderson, K. E., Kappas, A., & Conney, A. H. (1979). Stimulatory effect of brussels sprouts and cabbage on human drug metabolism. *Clinical Pharmacology and Therapeutics, 25*, 88–95.

Parker, L. (1984). A national tragedy: The task force that could not find hunger but found a block grant instead. *Health and Medicine, 2*(3), 7–11.

Parkin, D. M., Henney, C. R., Quirk, J., & Crooks, J. (1976). Deviation from prescribed drug treatment after discharge from hospital. *British Medical Journal, 2*, 686–688.

Passmore, R. (1964). Carbohydrates, the Cinderella of nutrition. In G. E. W. Wolstenholme & M. O'Connor (Eds.), *Diet and bodily constitution* (pp. 59–68). Boston: Little, Brown.

Patriarca, P. A., Kendal, A. P., Stricof, R. L., Weber, J. A., Meissner, M. K., & Dateno, B. (1983). Influenza vaccination and warfarin or theophylline toxicity in nursing home residents. *New England Journal of Medicine, 308*, 1601–1602.

Pearce, J. W., LeBow, M. D., & Orchard, J. (1981). Role of spouse involvement in the behavioral treatment of overweight women. *Journal of Consulting and Clinical Psychology, 49*(2), 236–244.

Personal papers: Obesity and sugar addiction. (1963). *Lancet, 1*, 768.

Pinto, J., Huang, Y. P., Pelliccione, N., & Rivlin, R. S. (1982). Cardiac sensitivity to the inhibitory effects of chlorpromazine, imipramine and amitriptyline upon formation of flavins. *Biochemical Pharmacology, 31*, 3495–3499.

Pinto, J., Huang, Y. P., & Rivlin, R. S. (1981). Inhibition of riboflavin metabolism in rat tissues by chlorpromazine, imipramine and amitriptyline. *Journal of Clinical Investigation, 67*, 1500–1506.

Pinto, J., Huang, Y. P., & Rivlin, R. S. (1985). Inhibition by chlorpromazine of thyroxine modulation of flavin metabolism in liver, cerebrum and cerebellum. *Biochemical Pharmacology, 34*, 93–95.

Plein, J. B., & Plein, E. M. (1981). Aging and drug therapy. *Annual Review of Gerontology and Geriatrics, 2*, 211–254.

Poikolainen, K. (1984). Estimated lethal ethanol concentrations in relation to age, aspiration, and drugs. *Alcoholism: Clinical and Experimental Research, 8*, 223–225.

Ray, W. A., Federspiel, C. F., & Schaffner, W. (1980). A study of antipsychotic drug use in nursing homes: Epidemiologic evidence suggesting misuse. *American Journal of Public Health, 70,* 485–491.

Reddy, B. S., Cohen, L. A., McCoy, G. D., Hill, P., Weisburger, J. H., & Wynder, E. L. (1980). Nutrition and its relationship to cancer. *Advances in Cancer Research, 32,* 237–345.

Reidenberg, M. M. (1977). Obesity and fasting: Effects on drug metabolism and drug action in man. *Clinical Pharmacology and Therapeutics, 22,* 729–734.

Reidenberg, M. M. (1982). Drugs in the elderly. *Medical Clinics of North America, 66,* 1073–1078.

Reidenberg, M. M., Levy, M., Warner, H., Coutinho, C. B., Schwartz, M. A., Yu, G., & Cheripko, J. (1978). Relationship between diazepam dose, plasma level, age, and central nervous system depression. *Clinical Pharmacology and Therapeutics, 23,* 371–374.

Resnick, L. M., Laragh, J. H., Sealey, J. E., & Alderman, M. H. (1983). Divalent cations in essential hypertension: Relations between serum ionized calcium, magnesium, and plasma renin activity. *New England Journal of Medicine, 309,* 888–891.

Reynolds, M. D. (1984). Institutional prescribing for the elderly: Patterns of prescribing in a muncipal hospital and a municipal nursing home. *Journal of the American Geriatrics Society, 32,* 640–645.

Riggs, B. L. Wahner, H. W., Dunn, W. L., Mazess, R. B., Offord, K. P., & Melton, L. J. III. (1981). Differential changes in bone mineral density of the appendicular and axial skeleton with aging: Relationship to spinal osteoporosis. *Journal of Clinical Investigation, 67,* 328–335.

Riley, M. W., & Foner, A. (1968). *Aging and society: An inventory of research findings.* New York: Russel Sage Foundation.

Risch, S. C., Groom, G. P., & Janowsky, D. S. (1981). Interfaces of psychopharmacology and cardiology: Part I. *Journal of Clinical Psychiatry, 42,* 23–34.

Rivlin, R. S. (1981). Nutrition and aging: Some unanswered questions. *American Journal of Medicine, 71,* 337–340.

Rivlin, R. S. (1982). Nutrition and cancer: State of the art. Relationship of several nutrients to the development of cancer. *Journal of the American College of Nutrition, 1,* 75–88.

Rivlin, R. S. (1983). Nutrition and the health of the elderly: A growing concern for all ages. *Archives of Internal Medicine, 143,* 1200–1201.

Roe, D. A. (1975). *Drug-induced nutritional deficiencies.* Westport, CT: AVI Publishing.

Roe, D. A. (1978). Diet-drug interactions and incompatibilities. In J. N. Hathcock & J. Coon (Eds.), Nutrition and drug interrelations (pp. 319–345). New York: Academic Press.

Roe, D. A. (1979). Interactions between drugs and nutrients. *Medical Clinics of North America, 63*(5), 985–1007.

Rosenbaum, E. H., Stitt, C. A., Drasin, H., & Rosenbaum, I. R. (1978 and 1980). *Health through nutrition: A comprehensive guide for the cancer patient.* San Francisco: Alchemy Books.

Rosner, B. A., & Cristofalo, V. J. (1981). Changes in specific dexamethasone binding during aging in W1-38 cells. *Endocrinology, 108,* 1965–1971.

Roth, G. S., & Hess, G. D. (1982). Changes in the mechanisms of hormone and neurotransmitter action during aging: Current status of the role of receptor and post-receptor alterations (review). *Mechanisms of Ageing and Development, 20,* 175–194.

Roth, H., Caron, H. S., & Hsi, B. P. (1971). Estimating a patient's cooperation with his regimen. *American Journal of Medical Sciences, 262,* 269–273.

Sambuy, Y., & Bittles, A. H. (1984). The effects of *in vitro* ageing on the exopeptidases of human diploid fibroblasts. *Mechanisms of Ageing and Development, 26,* 13–22.

Sapolsky, R. M., Krey, L. C., & McEwen, B. S. (1983). Corticosterone receptors decline in a site-specific manner in the aged rat brain. *Brain Research, 289,* 235–240.

Schaefer, A. E. (1982). Nutrition policies for the elderly. Proceedings of a symposium on nutrition and aging, Chicago, July 23–24, 1981. *American Journal of Clinical Nutrition, 36,* 819–822.

Schafer, L. C., Glasgow, R. E., McCaul, K. D., & Dreher, M. (1983). Adherence to IDDM regimens: Relationship to psychosocial variables and metabolic control. *Diabetes Care, 6,* 493–498.

Schiffman, S. (1977). Food recognition by the elderly. *Journal of Gerontology, 32,* 586–592.

Schlenker, E. D., Feurig, J. S., Stone, L. H., Ohlson, M. A., & Mickelson, O. (1973). Nutrition and the health of older people. In D. M. Watkin & G. V. Mann (Eds.), Symposium on nutrition and aging, part II. *American Journal of Clinical Nutrition, 26,* 1111–1119.

Schmandt, J., Shorey, R., & Kinch, L. (1980). *Nutrition policy in transition.* Lexington, MA: D. C. Heath.

Schmucker, D. L. (1984). Drug disposition in the elderly: A review of critical factors. *Journal of the American Geriatrics Society, 32,* 144–149.

Schmucker, D. L. (1985). Subcellular and molecular mechanisms underlying the age-related decline in liver drug metabolism. In R. N. Butler & A. G. Bearn (Eds.), *The aging process: Therapeutic implications* (pp. 117–134). New York: Raven Press.

Schocken, D. D., & Roth, G. S. (1977). Reduced beta-adrenergic receptor concentrations in ageing man. *Nature, 267,* 856–858.

Schulz, J. H., Carrin, G., Krupp, H., Peschke, M., Sclar, E., & Van Seenberge, J. (1974). *Providing adequate retirement income: Pension reform in the United States and abroad*. Hanover, NH: University Press of New England, for Brandeis University Press.

Schwartz, D., Wang, M., Zeita, L., & Goss, M. E. (1962). Medication errors made by elderly, chronically ill patients. *American Journal of Public Health, 52,* 2018-2029.

Scrimshaw, N. (1964). Ecological factors in nutritional disease. *American Journal of Clinical Nutrition, 14,* 112-122.

Seidl, L. G., Thornton, G. F., Smith, J. W., & Cluff, L. E. (1966). Studies on the epidemiology of adverse drug reactions, Part III: Reactions in patients on a general medical service. *Johns Hopkins Hospital Bulletin, 119,* 299-315.

Shaw, M. T., Spector, M. H., & Ladman, A. J. (1979). Effects of cancer, radiotherapy and cytotoxic drugs on intestinal structure and function. *Cancer Treatment Review, 6,* 141-151.

Shils, M. E. (1979). Nutritional problems induced by cancer. *Medical Clinics of North America, 63*(5), 1009-1025.

Shock, N. W. (1952). Age changes in renal function. In A. I. Lansing (Ed.), *Cowdry's problems of ageing* (3rd. ed., pp. 614-630). Baltimore, MD: Williams & Wilkins.

Shock, N. W. (1962). The science of gerontology. In F. C. Jeffers (Ed.), *Proceedings of seminars, 1959-1961* (pp. 123-140). Durham, NC: Duke University, Council on Aging and Human Development.

Shock, N. W. (1977). Systems integration. In C. E. Finch & L. Hayflick (Eds.), *Handbook of the biology of aging* (pp. 639-665). New York: Van Nostrand Reinhold.

Shock, N. W. (1982). The role of nutrition in aging. *Journal of the American College of Nutrition, 1,* 3-9.

Shock, N. W., Greulich, R. C., Andres, R., Arenberg, D., Costa, P. T. Jr., Lakatta, E. G., & Tobin, J. D. (1984). *Normal human aging: The Baltimore Longitudinal Study of Aging.* NIH Publication No. 84-2450. Washington, DC: U.S. Government Printing Office.

Shock, N. W., & Norris, A. H. (1970). Neuromuscular coordination as a factor in age changes in muscular exercise. In D. Brunner & E. Jokl (Eds.), *Medicine and sport, Vol. 4: Physical activity and aging* (pp. 92-99). Basel, Switzerland: S. Karger.

Shubik, P. (1979). Food additives (natural and synthetic). *Cancer, 43* (5 Suppl.), 1982-1986.

Shulman, N. (1975). Life-cycle variations in patterns of close relationships. *Journal of Marriage and the Family, 37*(4), 813-821.

Siegel, G. B. (1982). Drugs and the ageing. *Regulatory Toxicology and Pharmacology, 2,* 287-295.

Simonson, W. (1984). *Medication and the elderly: A guide for promoting proper use.* Rockville, MD: Aspen.

Slovik, D. M., Adams, J. S., Neer, R. M., Holick, M. F., & Potts, J. T. Jr. (1981). Deficient production of 1,25 dihydroxyvitamin D in elderly osteoporotic patients. *New England Journal of Medicine, 305,* 372–374.

Smale, A. H. (1979). Psychological aspects of anorexia: Areas for study. *Cancer, 43*(5 Suppl.), 2087–2092.

Smith, J. M., & Baldessarini, R. J. (1980). Changes in prevalence, severity, and recovery in tardive dyskinesia with age. *Archives of General Psychiatry, 37,* 1368–1373.

Spencer, H. (1982). Osteoporosis: Goals of therapy. *Hospital Practice, 17*(3), 131–148.

Spencer, H., & Kramer, L. (1985). Factors influencing calcium balance in man. In R. Rubin, G. Weiss, & J. Putney (Eds.), *Calcium in biological systems* (pp. 583–590). New York: Plenum.

Spencer, H., Kramer, L., DeBartolo, M., Norris, C., & Osis, D. (1983). Further studies of the effect of a high protein diet as meat on calcium metabolism. *American Journal of Clinical Nutrition, 37,* 924–929.

Spencer, H., Kramer, L., Lesniak, M., DeBartolo, M., Norris, C., & Osis, D. (1984). Calcium requirements in humans: Report of original data and a review. *Clinical Orthopaedics and Related Research, 184,* 270–280.

Spencer, H., Kramer, L., Norris, C., & Osis, D. (1982). Effect of small doses of aluminum-containing antacids on calcium and phosphorous metabolism. *American Journal of Clinical Nutrition, 36,* 32–40.

Spencer, H., Kramer, L., Osis, D., & Norris, C. (1978a). Effect of phosphorous on the absorption of calcium and on the calcium balance in man. *Journal of Nutrition, 108,* 447–457.

Spencer, H., Kramer, L., Osis, D., & Norris, C. (1978b). Effect of a high protein (meat) intake on calcium metabolism in man. *American Journal of Clinical Nutrition, 31,* 2167–2180.

Spencer, H., Kramer, L., & Osis, D. (1982). Factors contributing to calcium loss in aging. *American Journal of Clinical Nutrition, 36,* 776–787.

Spencer, H., Menczel, J., Lewin, I., & Samachson, J. (1965). Effect of high phosphorous intake on calcium and phosphorous metabolism in man. *Journal of Nutrition, 86,* 125–132.

Spencer, H., Rubio, N., Rubio, E., Indreika, M., & Seitam, A. (in press). Chronic alcoholism, a frequently overlooked cause of osteoporosis in males. *American Journal of Medicine.*

Spriet, A., Reiler, D., Dechorgnat, J., & Simon, P. (1980). Adherence of elderly patients to treatment with pentoxifylline. *Clinical Pharmacology and Therapeutics, 27*(1), 1–8.

Steel, K., Gertman, P. M., Crescenzi, C., & Anderson, J. (1981). Iatrogenic illness on a general medical service at a university hospital. *New England Journal of Medicine, 304,* 638–642.

Surwillo, W. W., & Quilter, R. E. (1964). Vigilance, age, and response-time. *American Journal of Psychology, 77,* 614–620.

Swift, C. G., Swift, M. R., Hamley, J., Stevenson, I. H., & Crooks, J. (1983). CNS effects of chronic benzodiazepine hypnotic ingestion in the elderly. *British Journal of Clinical Pharmacology, 16,* 217P–218P.

Thompson, J. S., Wekstein, D. R., Rhoads, J. L., Kirkpatrick, C., Brown, S. A., Roszman, T., Straus, R., & Tietz, N. (1984). The immune status of healthy centenarians. *Journal of the American Geriatrics Society, 32,* 274–281.

Thompson, T. L., Moran, M. G., & Nies, A. S. (1983). Psychotrophic drug use in the elderly. *New England Journal of Medicine, 308,* 134–138, 194–199.

Todhunter, E. N. (1976). Life style and nutrient intake in the elderly. In M. Winick (Ed.), *Nutrition and aging* (pp. 119–127). New York: John Wiley.

Triggs, E. J., Nation, R. L., Long, A., & Ashley, J. J. (1975). Pharmacokinetics in the elderly. *European Journal of Clinical Pharmacology, 8,* 55–62.

Twum-Barima, Y., Finnigan, T., Habash, A. I., Cape, R. D. T., & Carruthers, S. G. (1984). Impaired enzyme induction by rifampicin in the elderly. *British Journal of Clinical Pharmacology, 17,* 595–596.

Ullah, M. I., Newman, G. B., & Saunders, K. B. (1981). Influence of age on response to ipratropium and salbutamol in asthma. *Thorax, 36,* 523–529.

Upton, R. A., Williams, R. L., Kelly, J., & Jones, R. M. (1984). Naproxen pharmacokinetics in the elderly. *British Journal of Clinical Pharmacology, 18,* 207–214.

U.S. Department of Health, Education, and Welfare. (1972). *Ten-state nutrition survey, 1968–1970. V-Dietary.* DHEW Publication No. (HSM) 72-8133. Atlanta, GA: Center for Disease Control.

U.S. Department of Health, Education and Welfare Poverty Studies Task Force. (1976). *The measure of poverty, a report to Congress as mandated by the Education amendments of 1974.* Washington, DC: U.S. Department of Health, Education and Welfare.

U.S. Department of Health, Education and Welfare. (1977). *Health and nutrition survey I (HANES I).* DHEW Publication No. (HRA) 77-1310. Hyattsville, MD: National Center for Health Statistics.

U.S. Senate, Select Committee on Nutrition and Human Needs. (1974a). *Guidelines for a national nutrition policy.* Washington, DC: U.S. Government Printing Office.

U.S. Senate, Select Committee on Nutrition and Human Needs. (1974b). *National nutrition policy study, report and recommendations: II.* Washington, DC: U.S. Government Printing Office.

U.S. Senate, Select Committee on Nutrition and Human Needs. (1977).

*Dietary goals for the United States* (2nd ed.). Washington, DC: U.S. Government Printing Office.

U.S. Senate, Subcommittee on Long-Term Care of the Special Committee on Aging. (1976). *Drugs in nursing homes: Misuse, high cost, and kickbacks.* Washington, DC: U.S. Government Printing Office.

Veith, R. C. (1984). Treatment of psychiatric disorders. In R. E. Vestal, (Ed.), *Drug treatment in the elderly* (pp. 317-337). Sydney, Australia: ADIS Health Science Press.

Vesell, E. S. (1979a). The antipyrine test in clinical pharmacology: Conceptions and misconceptions. *Clinical Pharmacology and Therapeutics, 26,* 275-286.

Vesell, E. S. (1979b). Pharmacogenetics: Multiple interactions between genes and environment as determinants of drug response. *American Journal of Medicine, 66,* 183-187.

Vesell, E. S., & Page, J. G. (1968). Genetic control of drug levels in man: Antipyrine. *Science, 161,* 72-73.

Vesell, E. S., & Page, J. G. (1969). Genetic control of the phenobarbital-induced shortening of plasma antipyrine half-lives in man. *Journal of Clinical Investigation, 48,* 2202-2209.

Vestal, R. E. (1978). Drug use in the elderly: A review of problems and special considerations. *Drugs, 16,* 358-382.

Vestal, R. E., Norris, A. H., Tobin, J. D., Cohen, B. H., Shock, N. W., & Andres, R. (1975). Antipyrine metabolism in man: Influence of age, alcohol, caffeine and smoking. *Clinical Pharmacology and Therapeutics, 18,* 425-432.

Vestal, R. E., Wood, A. J. J., Branch, R. A., Shand, D. G., & Wilkinson, G. R. (1979). Effects of age and cigarette smoking on propranolol disposition. *Clinical Pharmacology and Therapeutics, 26,* 8-15.

Vestal, R. E., Wood, A. J. J., & Shand, D. G. (1979). Reduced $\beta$-adrenoceptor sensitivity in the elderly. *Clinical Pharmacology and Therapeutics, 26,* 181-186.

Wade, A. E., Norred, W. P., & Evans, J. S. (1978). Lipids in drug detoxification. In J. N. Hathcock & J. Coon (Eds.), *Nutrition and drug interrelations* (pp. 475-503). New York: Academic Press.

Wandless, I., & Davie, J. W. (1977). Can drug compliance in the elderly be improved? *British Medical Journal, 1,* 359-361.

Watkin, D. M. (1983). *Handbook of nutrition, health and aging.* Park Ridge, NJ: Noyes Publications.

Watkin, D. M. (1984, May). *The goal: Rectangularize survival; The objective: Change behavior.* Paper presented at the diamond anniversary of the Flavor and Extract Manufacturers Association of the United States, Marco Island, Florida.

Wattenberg, L. W. (1971). Studies of polycyclic hydrocarbon hydroxylases of the intestine possibly related to cancer: Effect of diet on benzpyrene hydroxylase activity. *Cancer, 28,* 99-102.

Welch, D. (1981). Nutritional consequences of carcinogenesis and radiation therapy. *Journal of the American Dietetic Association, 78,* 467-471.

Williams, M. E. (1984). Clinical implications of aging physiology. *The American Journal of Medicine, 76,* 1049-1054.

Williams, R. L. (1983). Drug administration in hepatic disease. *New England Journal of Medicine, 309,* 1616-1622.

Williamson, J., & Chopin, J. M. (1980). Adverse reactions to prescribed drugs in the elderly: A multicentre investigation. *Age Ageing, 9,* 73-80.

Wood, A. J. J., Vestal, R. E., Wilkinson, G. R., Branch, R. A., & Shand, D. G. (1979). Effect of aging and cigarette smoking on antipyrine and indocyanine green elimination. *Clinical Pharmacology and Therapeutics, 26,* 16-20.

Yancik, R. (1983). Frame of reference: Old age as the context for the prevention and treatment of cancer. In R. Yancik, P. P. Carbone, W. B. Patterson, K. Steel, & W. D. Terry (Eds.), *Perspectives on prevention and treatment of cancer in the elderly* (pp. 5-17). New York: Raven Press.

Yoshikawa, T. T. (1984). Aging and infectious diseases: State of the art. *Gerontology, 30,* 275-278.

Youngren, D. E. (1981). Improving patient compliance with a self-medication teaching program. *Nursing, 11*(3), 60-61.

Yudkin, J. (1963). Nutrition and palatability with special reference to obesity, myocardial infarction, and other diseases of civilization. *Lancet, 1,* 1335-1338.

# Index